PLANT-BASED DIET MEAL PLAN

A KICK-START GUIDE FOR BEGINNERS THAT HELP YOU TO ORGANIZE YOUR MEALS WITH HEALTHY RECIPES, PURIFY YOUR BODY AND ENERGIZE YOUR MIND JUST CHANGING BAD EATING HABITS.

Table of Contents

Introduction

Thank you for choosing my book. The following chapters will discuss the way in which you will benefit from the plant based diet by choosing to eat healthy, delicious recipes that will make it easy for you to lose weight and keep it off while living a healthier lifestyle.

Choosing to live a plant based lifestyle is one of the most important decisions you will ever make. Plant-based diets contain lots of fresh vegetables and fruits, along with nuts, seeds, and whole-grains. There are massive amounts of food just waiting for you to discover them and how delicious they really can be. And you will be leaving behind all of the saturated fats and other toxic substances that are holding back your health now.

It really should not be thought of as a diet plan or a manner of eating because deciding to 'go vegan' will affect all the parts of your life. It will dictate what you buy at the grocery store, where you go to eat out, and may even dictate who you decide to hang out with in your private life. But this is a decision that you are making to benefit your life.

So, let us take a journey together. I shall be your food guide, taking you through some of the most incredible plant-based and vegan recipes.

Research also shows that plant-based eating is related to healthy weight management, lower mortality risk, and lower heart disease risk. It is also related to hypertension prevention and treatment, high cholesterol, and lower risk of certain cancers.

Chapter 1: What Is a Plant-Based Diet

Plant diet is a term that comes from the English plant-based diet, which would have to be translated as a plant-based diet. It evokes obvious associations with veganism, but do these terms really mean the same thing?

Veganism is often understood as a whole lifestyle that includes the fight to reduce animal suffering, pro-animal activism, and attitudes associated with it. A plant-based diet is, in this respect, a much narrower concept, limited only to diet. There are a few minor differences. A plant-based diet does not have to be 100% plant-based. May allow small amounts of meat, fish or dairy products. However, veganism does not allow this possibility. On the other hand, the plant-based diet should be health-oriented and based on low-processed products, while veganism is not necessarily the case. Many vegans like to eat unhealthy products if they were prepared without the participation of animal components.

To sum up - the plant diet assumes that most calories come from plant products that are low-processed and composed in the diet so as to promote good health and may or may not be a vegan diet.

Pillars of plant nutrition for better health

1. Eat fully on plant foods Eating real food that grows from earth is the most important thing. Most likely, the reason people don't

eat enough plant-based food is that they still don't realize how strong plant nutrients are in maintaining our health.

Most people still feed on the flesh and products of other animals, not because there is something so natural, necessary or rational about it, but primarily because the major marketing share in supermarkets, stores, and food advertising are occupied by meat, animal, fast, processed and packaged products. Vegetable foods without salt, sugar, and refined fat still account for only a small percentage of the food industry's profits.

2. Plant foods to be whole Eating only plant food is not enough to stay healthy. Everyone is a complete organism made up of whole cells. That is why all of our cells need the most comprehensive food we can provide.

Whole plant foods mainly include fruits, vegetables, grains, and legumes in their least processed and natural state. Nuts and seeds are also part of an entirely plant-based diet, as are mushrooms (though not plants), spices, and all green leaves. Eating whole foods restricts or excludes processed and extracted substances such as extracted fats, sugars, and proteins. This means as much as possible without extracted oils, no added sugar, and artificial sweeteners, no superfood packets of powders, or protein shakes.

3. Carbohydrates should be at the base In addition to the need for whole foods, our cells need, above all, sufficient energy. The main source of energy in the human body is food, which, when

eaten, is broken down into its main nutrients - carbohydrates, fats, proteins, and water. Of these, it is the carbohydrates that make the cells draw on their glycogen supply, the fuel that makes our body's engine run at full speed.

4. Don't drink your calories Drinking them is one of the easiest ways to burn excess calories in your body.

We now know that a statistically significant number of people may be drinking between 800 and 1200 calories a day from morning coffee or distemper, from coca-cola, energy drinks, or cappuccino to work, from the beer with friends afterward, or a glass of wine before going to bed. The problem is, our brains don't even register those calories as calories. Like any other creature on the planet, one does not need to drink anything but water to be healthy. If you still want to drink coffee, drink it clean - no added sugar. If you make herbal tea, drink it without any additional sweetener. In just a few days, you will notice how much more saturated and fresh you will feel.

5. Move Proper nutrition is not the whole story when it comes to human health. Just as we need a balance between nutrients for the body to function most optimally, so do we need a balance between diet, movement, and other lifestyle-related factors.

In addition to the storage of nutrients in whole plant foods and herbs, exercise also plays a preventative role in protecting us from cardiovascular disease, hypertension, diabetes, obesity, osteoporosis, protecting us from colds, infections, and depression. Physical activity improves functions of blood circulation, lungs, skin and muscle tone, healing of wounds, and lowering of bad cholesterol.

Chapter 2: Myths to dispel about plant-based diet

Myth 1: The helpfulness of a plant-based diet does not have scientific proof.

The reality of the situation is that there are many studies conducted to prove the efficiency of a plant based diet. One of the main reasons why this myth persists is due to the fact that there are so many diet programs that claim to bring healthy changes in the lives of the people and end up not doing so. This makes people conscious about any new "food trend" that appears. In fact, let's look at this study conducted by the Cleveland Clinic where they discovered that people who stuck to a plant-based diet found themselves having really low cholesterol levels (Esselstyn, 2007).

Myth 2: People do not usually get the required amount of protein out of a plant-based diet.

Once again, this myth is present because of the fact that there are many people who still believe that they need meat to gain protein. However, the reality is that you can get all the proteins that you are getting from animal-based food out of a plant-based one. These days, there are many cultures that still believe that meat is one of the most important sources of proteins.

Myth 3: Having grilled or fried meat is completely okay. In fact, grilling is a healthy way to prepare it.

Both statements above are a variation of the same belief that it is okay to fry or grill lean meat. Some even say that grilling is a healthy form of preparing the meat. But those beliefs are not entirely supported by science. In fact, the opposite is true; when you fry or grill such a product at high heat, they release advanced glycation end (AGE) substances. They contribute greatly towards inflammation and oxidative stress, both of which cause damage to the liver, kidney, heart, and bones. Additionally, it will increase your chances of developing Alzheimer's.

Myth 4: When you prepare plant-based foods, you are consuming high amount of carbohydrates.

Not all the carbs that you consume are the same. Different foods provide different levels of carbs. There are a whole lot of recipes that allow you to control your diet and the nutrition that you would like to have. For example, if you would like to load up on essential fibers, you definitely can. Alternatively, you can change the ingredients in many of the recipes to fit your dietary requirements.

Myth 5: You are more likely to feel hungry because you depend on plant-based foods.

Most people think that plant-based diet involves eating salads for the most part. That is not true because when you are on a plant-based diet, you are working with different flavors and recipes. In fact, for many of the recipes, you take something that is already popular and add a plant-based twist to it. Such recipes can include spaghetti, lasagnas, and even tacos. (They are all given in this book!) If you look at the standard American diet, however, then you are going to notice that the foods that most people consume are high in calories and low in nutrients. In other words, they are eating more without getting the nutrition that their bodies require. All of this is affecting their health in the long term.

Chapter 3: Why follow this type of diet

Plants as a Medicine

Medicine has always been made using plants. It is therefore crystal clear that the plant-based diet can serve as medicines to our bodies.

You may find that when a person is unwell, a health expert may recommend eating a particular plant-based food. This is because plants have always had medicinal properties.

Diet-Related Diseases

Some of the diseases that are diet-related include;

Diabetes

Cancer

Cardiac arrest

Foods that Reduce Inflammation

If you already eat a fairly healthy diet, you will have no trouble incorporating these foods into your meals. In fact, you may already be enjoying them and just need a few tweaks to increase their presence in your meal planning. Some of the good foods that prevent and reduce chronic inflammation are as follows:

Omega 3 Fatty Acids

Omega 3 fatty acids are found in fish and fish oil. They calm the white blood cells and help them realize there is no danger, so they will return to dormancy.

Fruits And Vegetables

Most fruits and vegetables are anti-inflammatory. They are naturally rich in antioxidants, carotenoids, lycopene, and magnesium. Dark green leafy vegetables and colorful fruits and berries do much to inhibit white blood cell activity.

At least nine servings of fruits and vegetables each day are recommended. One serving is about a half-cup of cooked fruits and vegetables or a full cup if raw. The Mediterranean Diet, rich in fruits and vegetables, is often suggested to individuals suffering from chronic inflammation.

Protective Oils And Fats

Yes, there are a few oils and fats that are actually good for chronic inflammation sufferers. They include coconut oil and extra virgin olive oil.

Fiber

Fiber keeps waste moving through the body. Since the vast majority of our immune cells reside in the intestines, it is important to keep your gut happy. Eat at least 25 grams of fiber every day in the form of fresh vegetables, fruits, and whole grains. If that doesn't provide enough fiber, feel free to take a fiber supplement.

Flavor your food with spices and herbs instead of bad fats and unsafe oils. Spices like turmeric, cumin, cloves, ginger, and cinnamon can enhance the calming of white blood cells. Herbs like fennel, rosemary, sage, and thyme also aid in reducing inflammation while adding delicious new flavors to your food.

Healthy snacks would include a limited amount of unsweetened, plain yogurt with fruit mixed in, celery, carrots, pistachios, almonds, walnuts, and other fruits and vegetables.

Plants for Weight Loss

Obesity is considered to be an epidemic nowadays. Shockingly, more than 69 percent of adults in the United States are considered obese or overweight. Making changes in your diet and your whole lifestyle can lead to drastic weight loss when done properly. The impacts of these changes can be promising and long lasting. There are numerous studies that determined plant-based diet plans are very effective for weight loss.

The whole-food plant-based diet plan is rich in fiber and restricts processed foods while forbidding soda, refined grains, fast food, candy, and added sugars, making it ideal for weight loss. An overall assessment of 12 research studies found that people who followed plant-based diet plans lost more weight (2 kg less, in almost 18 weeks as compared to non-plant-based diet followers). Therefore a plant-based diet plan can also keep you from gaining weight.

Chapter 4: Benefits Of Plant-based Vegan Eating

More and more people each year make the decisions to change to a vegan lifestyle and way of eating. Veganism can improve your life in so many ways, such as giving you marvelous health benefits and putting less stress on the environment. The reasons why someone might choose to switch to a vegan lifestyle are many and very personal. Whether you are changing just the way you eat or you are deciding to forego using any type of animal product is totally your decision. This book will address the vegan way of eating and how it will help you to live the healthy life you have always wanted to live.

One of the healthiest ways to live is by following a vegan diet. The plant-based diet will contain vegetables, fruits, seeds, nuts, legumes, beans, and whole-grains. Since the vegan diet relies heavily on these plant-based staples, it is a healthy diet higher in fiber, phytochemicals, minerals, and vitamins than the average diet. The healthy vegan diet is also full of iron, magnesium, folic acid, and various vitamins, while they are also relatively low in cholesterol and saturated fats.

Here are some of the most important benefits that switching to a vegan diet will offer you.

You will be eating a diet that is rich in nutrients. In the typical Western diet, meat and animal products are usually the stars of the show. They do not have a place in the plant-based diet, so they will be eliminated. You will need to rely heavily on plant-based foods. These foods will give you a higher daily consumption of certain vital nutrients that you will get from your food. Eating a vegan diet will give you more antioxidants, fiber, and other beneficial plant compounds. The diet will be richer in folate, magnesium, potassium, and Vitamins A, C, and E. It will be important for you to base your meals on whole foods and not vegan alternative pre-packaged and fast food options because these are severely lacking in nutrients and will not provide the sufficient amounts of nutrition that you need.

A plant-based vegan diet can help you lose weight. Even when people consuming a plant-based diet eat until they are full, they can still lose weight because the calorie counts are lower for fruits, veggies, and whole-grains than they are for meat servings. Consider the following table:

Calories in one three-ounce chicken breast: 204

Calories in one three-ounce hamburger patty: 213

Calories in three ounces of green beans: 26

Calories in three ounces of peaches: 33

Calories in three ounces of oatmeal: 70

When your diet is made of plant-based foods like fruits, vegetables, and whole grains , you can eat until you are full and still not be consuming that many calories. Because of the foods that are eaten, the vegan diet has a natural tendency to reduce your intake of calories. This will automatically give you weight loss without the need to focus on cutting or counting calories.

Following a vegan diet can help you to lower your risk of heart disease. The vegan diet can benefit the health of your heart by significantly reducing those common risk factors that lead to heart disease, such as obesity. The vegan diet can also help to reduce cholesterol levels, blood sugar levels, and your overall blood pressure. All three of these are factors that contribute to the development of heart disease. Plant-based foods are naturally low in saturated fats and cholesterol while providing the good fats your body needs to function.

Reducing pain and inflammation is a benefit of the vegan diet. Plant-based foods contain compounds that will decrease the symptoms of inflammation and the effects of osteoarthritis, which is an inflammatory disease. As the compounds help to relieve inflammation, the diet itself will help you to lose weight, which is an added bonus because obesity will add to inflammation and the effects of osteoarthritis. Four pounds of extra pressure is put on the joints in the lower body with just one pound of excess body weight.

Certain cancers can be prevented by consuming a vegan diet. Eating seven portions of fresh vegetables and fruits each day may help to lower your risk of developing certain cancers. Lowering your consumption of animal products may reduce the risk of developing colon, breast, and prostate cancer. And legumes can help to reduce the risk of colorectal cancer. Fruits, vegetables, and whole-grains provide the fiber your body needs to cleanse itself of waste products. Seven servings each day may seem like a lot of food, but a serving of fruit is one small to medium piece or one cup, and a serving of vegetables is one-half cup.

Plant-based foods may improve kidney function and lower blood sugar levels. People who regularly follow a plant-based diet, like a vegan diet, usually have higher insulin sensitivity, lower blood sugar levels, and a significantly lower risk of developing Type 2 Diabetes. Your body produces insulin to move the blood sugar derived from the foods you eat into your cells to be used as energy. In obese people, the cells have stopped responding to the insulin so the excess blood sugar is stored as fat in the body. Reducing the number of calories will result in lower blood sugar levels, which will result in the cells being more sensitive to the call of the insulin and allowing the blood sugar to enter, reducing or eliminating the need to store it as fat.

The key to successfully switching to a plant-based diet, like the vegan diet, is careful planning. If your diet is going to be healthy for you, then you will need to consume the right kinds of foods that will give you the types and amounts of nutrition that your body needs. It is easy to get certain nutrients when your diet includes meat and dairy, but when you cut these out, then you will need to source out different ways to get the proper level of nutrition for your overall health.

Vitamin D – This is found naturally in fatty fish, cheese, egg yolks, and beef liver. These foods are not part of a vegan diet so you might need to look to other sources for your daily requirement of Vitamin D. Eating soy products, drinking fortified orange juice, or spending just ten to fifteen minutes in the sun each day will provide you with the Vitamin D your body needs.

Essential fatty acids – Problems that are related to brain health, such as depression and cognitive impairment, are related to a lack of dietary essential fatty acids. If you remove fish from your diet, then you are removing a natural source of Omega-3, which is an essential fatty acid your brain needs for good function. But these fats can also be found in seeds and nuts like walnuts, chia seeds, and flaxseed; and in plant-based oils like canola oil, soybean oil, and flaxseed oil. You can also add more collards, spinach, and kale to your diet.

Protein – We usually look to animal products for our sources of protein, but they are not the only source available to you. On a plant-based diet, your protein will come from lentils, chickpeas, soybeans, and tofu.

Iron – Egg yolks and red meat are the best sources of dietary iron, and these foods are high in dietary cholesterol. Fruits, tofu, and black-eyed peas are good sources of dietary iron. Quinoa, pumpkin seeds, spinach, and legumes are also good sources.

Vitamin B-12 – You will feel weak and tired if your body lacks this vitamin. It can be challenging for vegans to get enough Vitamin B-12 from their diets because it is not found in plants. You might either need to take a supplement or load up on soy drinks, fortified rice, and fortified cereals.

So knowing that you want to eat a more plant-based diet like the vegan diet and actually beginning to eat that way are two different things. Many people personally struggle with the idea of giving up animal products as part of their daily diets. After all, the typical Western meal is centered on some sort of meat dish. In many other countries, the meat is a side dish to the vegetable. Whether you just want to change to a more plant-based diet or move into a full vegan mode, there are things you can do to ease into a more plant-based diet that will make it easier for you to go fully vegan if you so desire.

The star of your meal are vegetables. Too often people think about what they are giving up, as in 'I am giving up beef' and not thinking about what they will be allowed to eat. Most people would not pair steak with pinto beans, but both are good sources of iron. If you don't eat the steak, then the pinto beans can become the main dish of the meal, and the beans will keep you fuller longer for fewer calories than the steak will.

Choose to eat a variety of whole-grains. If you change the white bread and white pasta in your diet to whole-grains like quinoa and brown rice, you will be eating extra fiber that will help you to lose weight. Also, quinoa and brown rice will add B vitamins and iron to your diet, where the white bread and pasta will not, as these essential items are stripped out during the refining process.

Always make good whole food choices. Vegan margarine on garlic bread is not any better for your heart than eating regular butter, and vegan cookies will expand your waistline just like regular cookies will. Never assume those food products that are labeled 'vegan' are healthier than their animal-product counterparts. These foods often contain coconut oil and palm oil, both of which are full of saturated fats. It is better to stick to nutritious whole foods that are vegan, like guacamole and whole-grain chips, dried fruit and nuts, or hummus with celery or carrots.

Make sure you get your vitamins from your food when possible. One vitamin that is often overlooked is Vitamin D because the typical Western diet will provide you with Vitamin D from yogurt, milk, and fish. On a more plant-based diet, you will need to spend some time in the sun every day, about ten minutes, or drink fortified non-dairy drinks such as orange juice, almond milk, or soy milk. Vitamin B-12 is also often overlooked because, in the Western diet, you get your amounts from dairy foods, eggs, poultry, fish, and meat. On a plant-based diet, a supplement may be needed. Vitamin B-12 can also be found in fortified energy bars and cereals.

Don't overlook your iron intake. Again, this is another nutrient that is readily found in the Western diet of chicken and red meat.

Iron is available in plant sources like leafy greens, legumes, and beans, but the iron from those sources is not as easily absorbed by the body as the iron that comes from animal sources. A good way to boost your body's absorption of iron from plant-based foods is to pair a food rich in Vitamin C, such as citrus food, with a plant food rich in iron. Tossing slices of mandarin oranges with a bowl of leafy greens is one delicious way to do this. Just remember to keep the calcium-rich foods on your menu away from this combination because calcium inhibits the absorption of dietary iron.

You will need Omega-3 fatty acids to promote good health. These are important for the health of your heart and brain and are found in great quantities in fatty fish. You will also be able to get them from foods like walnuts and flaxseed, and from soy products and canola oils. You might also need to consider a supplement.

Investigate the world of plant-based protein. Protein is readily available in animal sources like cheese and meat, but it brings with it high amounts of unhealthy saturated fats. There are numerous sources of protein from plant-based foods available for the vegan diet, like beans, chickpeas, edamame (soybeans), tofu, tempeh, and lentils. You can also get supplies of protein from pumpkin seeds, sunflower seeds, walnuts, and almonds. It is also an easy matter to get protein from whole-wheat pasta, oatmeal, nut butters, and quinoa.

Eat more whole-grains that will keep you full and fit. If you change out your refined grain foods like white bread and white pasta for more whole-grains , you will add more fiber, iron, and B vitamins to your daily diet.

Consume a variety of foods from all colors of the rainbow. Eating the rainbow is one of the newest ways that people are following to ensure that they are eating a well-balanced diet. It means adding foods to your diet, vegetables, and fruits, in all of the available colors so that you are adding in a variety of vitamins and minerals to your diet. Vegetables and fruits are full of water and fiber, and these two compounds will help you to feel fuller for longer periods and will also help rid your body of toxins through waste removal. Also, the colors that make the foods beautiful to look at are made naturally by compounds that are good for you, such as:

Red foods contain phytochemicals that fight cancer and heart disease and improve the quality of your skin

Yellow foods provide potassium, phosphorus, riboflavin, magnesium, folate, and fiber as well as Vitamins A, B-6, and C

Blue foods provide resveratrol and anthocyanins, both of which are powerful antioxidants

Orange foods support the health of your eyes as well as reducing blood pressure and cholesterol. They also help your joints and bones to be strong and healthy

Green foods help fight heart disease and diabetes by helping to fight obesity. They are full of fiber and antioxidants.

Adopting a more plant-based diet or even fully converting to a vegan diet is not difficult. You will need to make the personal choice of just how far you want to go with this. Will it be just adopting more of a plant-based diet or a full-on vegan lifestyle? The choice is yours. Just remember that when you are trying new foods, do so with an open mind but a bit of caution. Take a field trip to the local grocery store and look at all of the beautiful choices in the produce section. Some of these you may never have eaten and would like to try, and you should. But for some things, it may be better to source out a vegan restaurant or friend and try a dish that they have made before you take the item home and prepare it yourself. There is no need to take home a whole zucchini or eggplants if you do not like the taste because you will never eat it. Don't be afraid to experiment, but do begin with those vegetables, fruits, whole-grains , seeds, and nuts that you already know you like and build meals around those items. Then begin adding in new food items. You will be surprised at the endless variety now available in your food choices.

Chapter 5: What is a meal plan

One of the challenges that you are bound to face when coming up with a plant-based meal plan is balancing nutritional needs. In a real sense, very few people have the know-how and expertise to strike a balance on which foods to choose to come up with a well-rounded meal. This because they are generally intimidated with the requirements of coming up with a reliable plant-based meal plan way before they even begin.

Come to think of it; this process does not have to so intimidating. There are some new techniques you can learn from if you are looking at it from a perspective of a non-vegan diet or one who is used to having ready-made foods in the past. They have been handy for us in the past over the years of living as healthy vegetarians and have admittedly simplified our way of leading healthier lives for that matter.

Making a transition to a vegan life is noble. It is convenient to understand and plan your next course of action, which is capable of changing your lifestyle entirely for the better.

Why Meal Planning?

Initially, when you embark on a plant-based meal, planning might seem to be a little, of course, as compared to just getting into the kitchen and cooking up random meals. You will be tempted on numerous occasions only to throw down the gauntlet and go down this route. So, why should you even bother yourself on how to educate yourself on proper meal planning? It might bring you great joy and happiness in your life than you previously thought.

Some of these benefits may include:

• A hassle-free week

• Less time on the decision-making process and no more overthinking of meals

• More comfortable and cheaper shopping for grocery

• Easy to manage meal plans and healthy lifestyle

• You can quickly meet your nutritional needs

• You can also delve into new recipes without fear

• You can quickly come up with a weight loss plan

• Can enable you to discern what works best for you efficiently and lastly

• You can also be able to account for every ingredient and meals on hand

How to Plan

You can start by going for either fresh or frozen produce to add on to the varieties of starch at your disposal. It is always prudent to stock up some greens in the refrigerator, not forgetting a few tomatoes, cucumber, bell pepper, cruciferous vegetables, zucchini, eggplant, mushrooms, and cucumbers. You can also make it easy for yourself by choosing the things you like the most, in addition to what is readily available at your disposal. One better option you can choose from is frozen, bananas, dates, apples, or oranges.

Chapter 6: How eliminate bad eating habits

Cooking is all about preparing food that best suits you with the rest of the family. We all cook food for different reasons or rather goals. Some objectives are good, while others might sound vague, but all in all, we all cook with one primary purpose of improving our health. We all try our best to make different plans for doing our kitchen work. It also becomes vital to make sure that everything comes out in its perfect order with enough tastes and flavors. Sometimes we go for taste and forget that the nutrients content also matters a lot, especially when our health is considered.

Our health has been a significant factor in many situations. Therefore, that's why we prefer to deal with anything affecting it, by all means, using different ways. We are more inclined to health issues when types of food we are preparing have been put into significant consideration. As has been said earlier, health is a factor of life, and when we fail to consider it, then we are doomed. Many people have so far inclined to fast foods that are being offered within the restaurant. These types of food referred to junk foods, and most of them have got a higher level of meat as a single ingredient. They are preferred due to their quick or natural mode of preparation.

In many cases, this occurs without knowing that some food such as meat, if not well cooked, will accelerate the thriving conditions of the internal worms. These warms include tapeworms that have severe complications with the internal body organs. These people have beliefs that the best restaurants within the world have been reserved for some high-class personality. This is just a belief since anyone with enough resources can visit those high-end restaurants. But these restaurants are served meat-related foods that have severe complications within the long run. Even though we are much aware of this, many argue that they lack time to prepare plant-based meals. That being creative enough to play with the plant-based recipes are time-consuming.

This has eventually affected the lives of many. Many have got health issues that hinder them from being productive in their capacity or even at work. These health issues include cancer-related complications, especially within the colon, breast, and even prostate cancer. Obesity has been another health issue over the years now. Many studies have been carried out on the possible ways to control these health issues, and many findings have narrowed down to plant-based cooking.

It is, therefore, possible for all of us to look for critical ways to understand plant-based food and how we can embark on it. Understanding plant-based cooking will even make you better and start making or preparing excellent plant-based meals, which are delicious and yummy. This knowledge will also help you in indulging in this kind of diet that you have never belonged to. Over some time, your cooking skills will improve, and having these basics; you will never require additional time or effort to prepare this food. You will be ultimately an experienced guru in the field of cooking plant-based meals without following even the recipes.

The plant-based cooking or preparation of food can be precisely defined as the type of cooking which involves or revolves around food prepared from plants. This implies that your diet will have more plant food as compared to other kinds of food. In other words, your food will be more of plant sources than meat and sometimes will even have no traces of meat at all — these diets composed of nuts, legumes, beans, whole grains and much more.

Apart from that, the nutrition recommendation also covers almost all types of vitamins. These meals have higher levels of fiber. They also contain other types of nutrients needed within the body. This type of cooking also offers enough minerals that are helpful in the optimal healthy life of a person, thus leading to a long lifespan. They also and also act as a preventive mechanism towards different diseases or infections. These diseases arise from heart complications and involve coronary thrombosis and other blood-related disorders such as blockage of blood vessels and much more. These types of food comprise of vegetables and fruits which have red, orange and yellow colors such as carrots, tomatoes, mangoes and much more. The same also includes green vegetables such as spinach, kales, romaine lettuce, broccoli, bok choy, among others. Traces of leeks, onions and even garlic can also be regarded as part and parcel of phytonutrient.

Plant-based cooking has more to offer in terms of disease curbing. As usual, this is compared to a vegetarian diet. The same meal plan is also compared to the Mediterranean diet even though the latter two have been found to support the health issues. This also leads us to an urge to understand these differences to be able to comprehensively understand what we shall be doing in the kitchen when preparing plant-based dishes.

The Mediterranean diet has its initial roots from plant-based sources and also incorporates other foods like fish, yogurt, poultry, and so on. Things such as meat and sweets are offered in fewer quantities even though not very often. This Mediterranean diet has been inclined to the positive side of our health. Studies have shown that the risk of getting heart diseases have reduced tremendously. There is a decreased level of metabolic syndrome with a good number of people showing a reduction in the level of health issues arising from this syndrome. Cases like cancers have also reduced.

This diet was found to be of help to people suffering from cancerous diseases such as colon, prostate, and even breast cancer. With this diet, if well offered, the frailty in older people will reduce too. This diet can also help to improve the functionality of your brain and physical body in general. However, this diet is slightly different from a vegetarian diet.

A vegetarian diet is gotten purely from plant-based meals. The same meal is also harvested from cooking meals with the plan in mind. Currently, only a few people are taking additional dietary supplements.

Vitamin B12 is one of these supplements. It's used to help their consumers in acquiring all the nutrients needed by their bodies. The vegetarian diets come in handy in different forms or rather types. It's now upon you to choose the best that fits you and the rest of your family. It is good to understand that your health issues should give you a direction when it comes to choosing the type of vegetarian food. There are different types which include a semi-vegetarian diet. This type consists of eggs, products of dairy, meat but not always, seafood, fish, and even poultry. A different kind of vegetarian diet is a pescatarian. It also includes eggs, it has fish in it, has seafood and some dairy products. However, this diet lacks meat or poultry. The last type though not often is called lactose vegetarian diet, which comprises using eggs and dairy foods only. This implies that this diet does not entertain anything to do with meat, fish, poultry, or even seafood.

Another related plant-based diet is the Nordic diet. This diet has some features similar to the Mediterranean cooking plan. It also has a high level of whole grains and berries. Other meals that you can look at include fatty fish such as salmon and so on. There are also vegetables, fruits, and even legumes. This diet also contains eggs and some dairy products with a high limitation of red meat and other processed foods. It does not involve sweets too.

The human race is funny when it comes to choosing between a diet comprising of meat in abundance supply and the one which has plant-based sources. It is now clear that many people eat meat not because of its nutritional value but because of its taste. They have forgotten that flavor and nutrition cannot go hand in hand. They are always going into different directions. The same implies that it will take some more time to instill this kind of information into the current generation. For them to digest it, they will still need much more time. And as a result of this, many will suffer from health-related diseases.

Many people argue that the actual plant-based cooking plan has no dairy and its products, that they have no meat at all or even oils and eggs. Many seem not to understand the difference that has been stipulated above concerning vegetarian diets, Mediterranean food, and even Nordic dishes. Others go ahead to hardening of the blood vessels such as arteries which later lead to heart disease.

Again there are a lot of talks that cover the consumption of eggs and meat. In the opinion of such individuals, the incorporation and their intake lead to the thriving of cancerous cell multiplication. It's now clear that many people have had a severe misconception about foods like oils. Surprisingly, to some point, they are not aware of the sources of these oils to be from plants like sunflower, avocados, canola, or even olives.

We are much obsessed with the word "plant" without taking much consideration, the word "plant-based." And, in this scenario, many argue that dairy products even if offered in fewer quantities, will still have various side effects on the body. This is true based on the knowledge that these fewer quantities are critical supplements in the building of muscles. Apart from that, the meals also lower blood pressure. This low quantity also helps in the reduction of tooth decay, reduces obesity, and also can help in the prevention of cancer.

Many people have argued that diet is perfect for your health. However, when it comes to discussing some of the issues affecting our bodies, the results have been overwhelming towards the plant-based meals. The idea is based on the fact that it can quickly help in curbing and controlling many diseases.

A group of scholars, however, argued that, even though plant-based meal plans are best for our diets, not all should be preferred. Their study found that the best plant-based meal plans are those who emphasized on ingredients that are fresh and whole. And due to this, they cautioned on the use of processed plant foods like fully refined maize flour, fully refined wheat flour and so on. As a result, they argued that when all these are observed, then the issue of health will be solved a notch higher. All these are meant to help us understand the plant-based cooking and their benefits. Understanding the plant-based diet plan can be a cumbersome task, especially when you have a family who hates fruits and vegetables. The only way to go about it is to show them the source of food.

It's also vital to discuss the side effects of the food on the body. Besides, it's essential to provide good reasons why the best options for cooking are embracing organic meals and natural cooking meals. Giving a clear view on why some foods are better than others will at least help them to understand the plant-based cooking. Also, having that passion and love boosts the morale of adopting plant-based sources of food. Below is a detailed summary of the benefits of plant-based cooking, especially after having a comprehensive review of the plant-based dish.

The first benefit of understanding plant-based cooking is that it will help us in restoring our health and curbing of diseases. Many studies have proved beyond doubts that focussing on the plant-based cooking plan helps a lot in returning our healthy initial condition or rather situation. This involves the entire use of these meals in our daily diets. Diseases like cancer, especially cancer of the colon, prostate cancer, and even breast cancer, have been found to have a negative result with the plant-based foods. This implies that the cancerous cells are entirely affected by the presence of this food within the body system. As a result, their day to day thriving or growing is diminished and may even fail to show up. Due to this, the effect of cancer reduces, and those already diagnosed can also get healed.

Again, people who are mainly into this diet are not risky in cases or issues touching disease. Therefore they will never be prone to this disease. Following this diet will tremendously reduce heart-related conditions such as coronary thrombosis, arteriosclerosis, and so on. This leads to enough flow of blood within the blood vessels and with the required pressure. As a result, cases of heart attack will be nothing to worry about. We have other kinds of blood-related diseases such as elephantiasis which come as a result of poor blood circulation within the lower organs of the body, especially the limbs. Well, observation and considering this diet will help us to eliminate this.

Understanding of plant-based food or meal plans can also help us in improving our way of eating. The idea refers to eating habits. We are coming from a rigid society obsessed with much technology that doesn't allow us to concentrate on plant-based food. This over obsession, especially on fast food such as junks and the rest, has misled us to channel our way to poor eating habits.

With the help of this handbook, we can improve our eating habits. With that said, excellent plant-based meal plans have an accurate idea of what to eat and when to it. The same implies that the meal has specified breakfast, lunch as well as supper. At the same time, snacks and dinner have been organized categorically.

We are living in a world where taste seems to be better than nutrition. A good number of people eat junk foods, especially meat just because of how these food taste and not their value. This leads to a high level of build-up fats within the muscles and walls of the stomach. Unhealthy eating habits later result in obesity and other health-related diseases. By understanding the benefits of plant-based cooking, we get the chance to meet a world free from excess unhealthy meals such as junk food. The case also implies that the level of meat-related disease is reduced. Plant-based diets eliminate all these thus making us lead a good and a better life.

Our understanding of plant-based food or rather meal plans help us to decrease in weight. That's losing weight. Plant-based cooking relies mainly on foods that have their sources from plants. These types of foods include vegetables like kales, spinach, broccoli, and much more. This diet also contains fruits like mangoes, tomatoes, lettuce, and so forth. Cereals such as wheat, maize flour, oats, and much more are also part of this.

When plant-based cooking plans are fully understood and followed, health sectors within the society or a community improves. Lots of medications become a past tense thing. The people live a happy life. The immune system of everyone increases and falling sick diminishes. As a result, drugs become eliminated or somewhat reduced to a minimal level. The same instance will lead to a rise in the economy within the community since not much will be spent on medication. This is made possible by the help of a careful comprehension of plant-based cooking. An excellent plant-based diet also has fewer complications within the body as compared to the diets full of meat and other fatty foods. And due to this, there is no build-up of disease within the body tissues that will eventually require medications.

Knowledge of plant-based cooking if fully implemented can help us eradicate cruelty within the world, thus making the sustainability of the world to be more manageable. Chaos and cruelty always come as a result of sheer misunderstanding within different sectors. This is the same for even health sectors. Maintaining good health is the main objective of our daily lives, and without doing this, then the world will be full of chaos.

Imagine a world where the health sector is below standards. This implies that many people will be suffering from diseases such as heart attacks plus other blood related or heart-related diseases. This will eventually leave many industries with fewer people in terms of employees. Competent personnel within the ranks of the company will reduce, and obesity increases. All these will create cruelty and chaos that will be hard to eradicate. In a situation where the knowledge of this diet is well understood, then the correct implementation is followed, chances of cruelty become low. This makes the world to be easily manageable.

This type of diet always saves time. Also, its preparation is based on cooking using the purest forms of recipes. The result is you enjoying a healthy diet. Additional cooking and meal preparation plans don't involve complicated methods that take time to understand. All the skills required to make these recipes are easy to acquire. The duration of cooking is also less since they take the shortest time possible to get prepared. This leads to saving of your precious time that can be invested in other productive responsibility within the community or in an organization. Understanding the plant-based cooking diet will eventually allow us to be more productive in other areas since preparations of these foods require less time.

These types of food from plant-based sources require less fuel. A less or little amount of energy will often be used in their preparations. As a result, energy is saved. When this occurs, the high energy levels lead to a better economy. The world economies grow and thrive well. A good economy is characterized by good governance. Apart from that, the people comprising that economy will lead a better life. The result is usually courtesy of our well comprehensive nature towards our plant-based cooking.

Another beneficial side of observing and understanding the plant-based cooking plans is that this diet increases longevity. It has been observed that those who indulge in plant-based foods live longer in that they have a longer lifespan. During this period, they are always healthy and can even do hiking. The increase in life span is due to the preferable diet. The diet consists of whole grains, vegetables, fruits such as mangoes, tomatoes, and even other types of food such as onions, garlic. This diet also lacks excess meat and has a high content of fiber and moderate fats. This implies that the person consuming all these will have a healthy body. His immune system becomes stronger and stronger and chances of getting illness are minimal. This person will live a better healthy life that's free from sickness or any diseases. It's clear to note that the same will eventually lead to an increase in lifespan. Also, this is only made possible by the help of the knowledge gotten from plant-based cooking plans.

Plant-based meal plans have several options to choose from. A good understanding of plant-based cooking will enable you to choose from different types of plant sources. By planning your meals, you will be able to avoid cooking the same classes of food. In this case, you shall avoid making the same meals as in your initial diets.

With the meal plan in your mind, you have got a wider or an extensive collection of fruits, vegetables, and grains. You can go greens sometimes by choosing large varieties such as kales, spinach and so on. You can choose other types of fruits, such as apples, oranges, tomatoes, and many others. You can have your breakfast served in whole grains by going for oats and so on. So, in this plant-based meal plan, you will be in a position to even enjoy your food. The fact is appended to the foundation of the health benefits of such meals. It doesn't have boredom of cooking the same type of food over and over again. This will also boost your kitchen morale, and always you will spend much of your time cooking these meals. When confidence has been raised, loving your food becomes easier; thus indulging becomes a soft spot in your diet.

No additional energy or effort is added or required in cooking plant-based meals, especially when a sound knowledge has been instilled in you about these types of food. The result is a beneficial factor here. It is easy to learn and master the skills needed, and you need no classroom in cooking plant-based meals. What you need here is your time and your love and likeness towards this diet.

These two factors should act as a tip to safeguard you and guide you on your way to preparing these meals. The only thing you need hereafter understanding the necessary knowledge in plant-based diets is the experience. Experience is all about cooking these recipes over some time. The move won't be an issue here since it will act as a driving force that will eventually help you to even crave for cooking these recipes daily. By doing so, your level of expertise will increase. You may also find it easy to make better meals compared to professionals.

Chapter 7: How plan the meals so diet works

It's is not easy to make a change in any diet that you quickly embrace. The decision to take on a plant-based meal plan is based on wanting to live healthier lives. The change might be inevitable later on after many realizations of what we get when we eventually abandon what we prefer to consume.

Changing from regular life diets to start incorporating plant-based foods will meet some resistance at first if not well understood. It is now through this that we have come up with different tips to follow to start a plant-based diet. These several tips can help us and make our understanding much more comfortable when dealing with plant-based foods. These tips also are used as guidelines that will help us not only today but even in the coming generations.

The first tip is all about setting rules and making sure that you are being initiated to new recipes of plant-based meals even twice a week. Regulations created by yourself will be quickly followed as compared to the ones formed and forced on you. In this plant-based diet, it is all about loving what you are doing. The created recipes will always be easy to follow, and once mastered, you will only be improving on them. One rule that can be created here is the setting of a day. This day is preserved mainly for one purpose, and that's making a plant-based meal.

Make it to the family and get their ultimate reviews on what you have done. Ask them to comment on the tastes and the food in general. The result will help you a lot, especially in your next meal.

The next tip here is all about creating a constant tendency towards plant-based meals. Make a plan for cooking this food more often within a week. Don't wait for ages to pass since you are getting induced to starting your plant-based diet. Practice makes perfect, and within a long time, your skills, especially necessary skills, will improve. Your experience will be a notch higher, and this will be reflected in your habits. Making cooking of plant meals frequent is one of the most excellent tips in jump-starting your plant-based meal. Along the way, you will get adapted to it. You'll also realize that you've changed your approach to how you always think of other types of food, such as diets full of meat and junk foods.

It's vital to grab recipes from the shelves or drawers where they are kept and reading. The habit can occur without necessarily making or preparing these foods. At the same time, the pattern can improve your skills and give you several tips and morale to embark on preparation later on. Reading equips one with the required skills and creativity needed in an area of expertise. After having enough knowledge and comprehension, especially on these plant-based recipes, you can now embark on that kitchen work. Follow your recipes slowly by slowly and get used to it after some trials. The action will make it even easier. You will start enjoying it, and without knowing, you will be in an excellent position to begin migrating from your current diet to plant-based diets.

Most of us usually use vegetables in our daily diets without knowing their value. They may also use the plants in meal preparation without having a rare view of what they do in our food. Some use vegetables because others have been using while some will try to incorporate it just because it is there. It is just well for your understanding about this, but if you want to jump-start into this diet, then go for the vegetables that people regard as unusual.

The ones that you have never used ever since you were born. The ones you have never even seen. Visit different fruits vendors store and have these unusual collections. Ask questions if in case you do not understand. Pick them and try using them already to check on their flavors and tastes. Your ability to pick the right plant-based meal plan will help you to choose which to use and not to use. It is good to note that these unusual vegetables can be used to compensate for flavors gotten from meat-related dishes. This choosing of particular types of plants is a good tip to start your plant-based diet.

As a beginner in this diet, the best tip for starting a plant-based diet meal plan will be, to begin with, vegetables. Try as much as possible to eat vegetables. The act can be during lunch and dinner or rather a supper. Make sure that your plate is always full of plants of different categories. Different colors can help you choose the different types you want to get to learn. Vegetables too can also be eaten as snacks, especially when combined with hummus or salsa. You can also use guacamole too in this combination and rest assured you will love it.

People eat meat, and it has been part and parcel of their daily diet. As said earlier, many prefer meat due to its taste. They don't go for it because of its nutritional value. In many cases, we can look for ways to change our thinking about meat. If we can all agree to reduce the level of intake of meat, our lives would be better. The reason is appended to the health benefits of taking vegetables and not meat.

Then, the same can be replaced with the high intake of the plant-based meal, and then we shall rest assured that at long last our thinking about meat will have to change. For us to improve our diet, then we need to know the side effects of taking meat in large quantities. One of the most dangerous side effects is its ability to build up within the body tissues. Together with fatty oils, your body loses shape and obesity will encroach. Life-threatening problems start arising, and this will only land you into the hospital as you seek medication. In the long run, your life will be affected by the economic challenges appended to it. As you realize you have wasted many resources in dealing with a condition, you could have controlled from the beginning. The action might cause some depression and stress. It's good to note that you are not supposed to withdraw all meat at once. In this case, you can change your approach towards meal intake.

Reducing the level of consumption will help us to indulge in plant-based cooking meals plan. You can also use this meat as just a side dish. That's like garnish. Avoid using meat as a centerpiece.

The types of fats and oils being used should be highly considered. Well-Chosen fats or oils will come from avocados, olive oil, some specific seeds and even nuts like groundnuts and so on. By doing this, you will be in a high position of being initiated to plant-based cooking.

As we all know, changing from one diet to another diet will be challenging. The case is specific, especially within a short period. What you need to do is to cook at least twice, thrice or even once within a week. Cook some plant-based food once or twice a week depending on how you might want.

You will learn how to jump-start your initiation period. You'll also understand what it takes to grasp the basic knowledge of plant-based meal planning.

In most cases, try to use more vegetables, beans, and even whole grains. Never use processed foodstuffs like processed and refined flour since this has got fewer nutrients and mostly lacks enough fiber needed within the body.

Another tip that will help you in starting a plant-based diet meal is by using whole grains during breakfast. Use it in high quantities since it will help you in adopting this kind of diet within a short period. It is not always easy to use all of these whole grains. The best way forward is to choose meals that can suit you and the rest of your family at first. Good examples will be highly recommended. These might include oats, barley, or even buckwheat. Here, you can add some flavors provided by different types of nuts and several seeds. Don't forget to include fresh fruits next to your reach.

Greens are some of the best vegetables preferable in the plant-based diet. They are also crucial in helping you to maintain a healthy diet. And going for them will help you jump start your long journey in embracing plant-based foods. Greens can be used at different levels and embracing it at the initial level is the best. Go for greens such as kales, spinach, collards and much more.

Another way to get induced to a plant-based diet is by using diets that revolve or contains salad. You can make the salad greens from leafy greens like spinach, romaine and sometimes the red leafy greens are preferred. Different kinds of vegetables are added here. These vegetables are added together with beans, peas, or even fresh herbs.

The best thing with fruits is that fruits can be consumed at any time and in any way. They don't have any form of rigid procedure or protocol that needs to be followed as far as their consumption is concerned. Eating fruits every day as dessert will help you get adapted to it. This will create some sorts of habits within you and without realizing you will be fully indulged in a plant-based meal.

Fruits play different roles in our diet plans. By consuming them every day, we can quickly boost our immunity. The same meals will help us to forget to focus more on eating healthy for the rest of our lives. For example, some fruits will help you reduce the level of craving for sugary sweets, especially after having the main meal. Fruits such as watermelon and apples can help in keeping hydrated. Therefore, you will be able to get used to it. Within the long run, you will be adapted to plant-based diet meals.

Another way that can also help you start your meal plan is by having curiosity or instead of being extra curious. Many studies have solid proof of interest as a tip in starting plant-based meal plans. Sometimes in life, you want to venture into something you never knew. You want to do something that you have not been doing, especially when it comes to cooking different meal plans.

Many times people have been obsessed with junk food and other meat-related foods. Trying something new is just out of curiosity and may take a reasonable period to understand fully. In the long run, you will develop skills that will eventually help you to do every work within the kitchen. As has been said earlier, changing from your healthy diet to a plant-based diet is not simple. However, after an extended period, you will be in an excellent position to embrace it. This comes about after your curiosity to do something new every day. You will get used to it over time.

Sometimes you can jump-start this plant meal as a result of love. Many people are trying something new. If you have that love for plant-related dishes, then you will be in an excellent position to embrace it after some time. The move will help you manage your eating habits.

Embracing plant-based diet meal plans will come in handy with the broader choice of the food sector to choose from. You will have an alternative source of food in addition to what you have been consuming over the last years. Having led by your love to eat plant-based meals or rather to change the diet will vastly help you to get used to it.

Within the long run, you will get familiarized and used to it. You will then start practicing it in your daily routines, thus reducing your urge on meat-related meals. For this one to work better, you must love eating too. The eventual result is just an aspect of life that will accelerate your objective in starting plant-based diet meal plans.

Another tip is about pairing foods. You can use this tool to have more excellent knowledge of which types of plant-based foods can be matched and results in good taste. You can do this pairing by combining several flavors. The result should give you a strong feeling that works for you.

The same is appended to the fact that trial and error works. When you comprehend food pairing completely, rest assured that your cooking skills and love of it are moving to the next level. The later will even enable you to cook your plant-based meal without checking or following your recipes. You shall also experience timely results in time reduction and saves energy too. Sometimes you need also to compare notes on different books about plant-based recipes and pick only the best that can help you begin on this.

You can choose a paper having a Mediterranean diet and another one having vegetarian food recipes or you can also go for the Nordic diet. Compare the notes and pick the similarities. The actions will make you understand much more about plant-based food and how to adequately prepare them. These books done by different authors will also help you with some inspiration and ideas on different flavors.

Watching is also regarded as another tip, which will help you to start plant-based meal plans. Have those videos concerning cooking at your reach. Several stations are dealing with cooking. Spend much time watching them as you dearly take notes. Make a date with your television and watch those food networks that talk much about plant-based diets.

Many studies have concluded that cooking videos are essential tools, especially in cooking. This is because, in your mind, you will be in a position to know how the food will look like even if you are not cooking. Using videos create some perfection in the kitchen. You'll have no stress or pressure here. It is all about watching and doing the required practice. Practicing now and then gives you that experience you need and will later help you to get embraced to the plant-based diet.

Chapter 8: Do I become vegan or vegetarian following this diet?

Plant-Based Vs. Vegan & Vegetarian

In some major ways, vegetable-based diets are different from vegan or vegetarian diets. First, let me explain the distinction between vegans and vegetarians: Lacto-Ovo vegetarians consume dairy and eggs, while vegans avoid all animal products and generally avoid the purchase, use, and use of animal products. Vegans and vegetarians that eat foods that are refined packaged, and may not even end up eating a healthy diet.

People on a herbal diet, by contrast, eat whole foods as close as possible to nature - vegetables, fruits, nuts, seeds, and the like. Someone on a plant-based diet may choose to eat vegan or vegetarian and may or may not use animal products. Some people on a generally vegetable-based diet may consume some animal products, but comprise a very small portion of their diet.

You have seen many people do it and talk about it. In fact, it seems that once someone gets into the plant-based diet, they don't not talk about it.

However, what exactly does it mean to adopt a plant-based diet? Do we have to head into the woods, find a tree, pull some leaves, and sauté them with salt and pepper? Hardly.

The confusion happens because we often break foods into various macronutrients, such as proteins, fats, and carbohydrates. At this point, we begin to compare various foods and see how we can curb different unnecessary nutrients from our diet. We hope to live to eat the best version of the things that we are currently living on.

Plant-based diet can vary from one person to another. However, the foundational idea is that we try to avoid processed food as much as possible and choose to use what we receive from the beautiful planet that we live in. By that, I mean the incredible ingredients derived from the earth. In essence, plant-based diet comes with a few benefits.

• Plant-based diet avoids using processed foods as much as possible.

• There are no animal products in the diet.

• The categories that are majorly included are vegetables, fruits, seeds and nuts, legumes, whole grains, and herbs and spices.

• The diet tries to limit the use of sugar, wheat-flour, and oil as much as possible.

• It focuses on the quality of food, mostly utilizing locally or farm-produced organic foods An important thing to remember here is that there are minimally processed foods included in the plant-based diet, such as non-dairy milk, tofu, and whole-wheat paste, to name a few. Overall, we aim to keep processed foods where they belong: on supermarket shelves, not in our refrigerators.

When people look at the list of foods that come in a plant-based diet, they are often focused on how little we have to work on. However, that is probably due to the fact that many of the meat options have suddenly been removed. It feels as though a major part of the diet has been excluded due to it. How can life be fun without a nice steak? What can we do without chicken wings? Is there anything that can be done without a delicious fish?

In reality, there are numerous ingredients that you can work with (which we shall see later). Additionally, the fun is not just in the ingredients but how we prepare them. With the demand for plant-based goods increasing around the world (Forgrieve, 2018), there are so many ways in which you can enjoy a wonderful meatless meal. The growing demand has seen a rise in people trying out new recipes and mashing up ingredients in interesting ways. Have you heard of smoothies that contain cayenne pepper? Sounds pretty exciting, doesn't it? We are going to look at such wonderful and delicious recipes along with so many more dishes that use wholesome and natural ingredients.

The thing is, you might also be averse to certain ingredients. For example, you might not be too fond of tofu or soy. That is alright. The best part about whole-food, plant-based diet is that you have so many ingredients to work with (literally the entire A to Z of awesome stuff available from nature). You are not picking it up to be forced to eat something. The main idea is to follow the diet. What kind of natural ingredients you use is entirely up to you.

Cutting Back on Animal-Based Foods

It's not easy to give up on sausages and fried chicken when they have been part of our diet for a long time. Some people experience withdrawals and get sudden cravings for meat.

There is a good reason why people are so hooked on to meat.

• Think of the marketing techniques of the meat industry. You are more likely to find an advertisement for a juicy burger or new steak joint than any information about vegetarian food.

• There is a lot of misconceptions about where we should get our nutrients from. For example, according to the World Health Organization (n.d.), we need at least 10% to 15% of protein in our diet; otherwise, we will start craving for it. Now, most people think that they can gain these proteins only from meat, and this myth has persisted for a long time. Hence, you may have heard someone recommend including meat in your diet in order to gain the 'missing' proteins. However, there are numerous plant sources for that. Nature has it all, after all.

• Human beings have a natural tendency to have fatty foods in their diet. In fact, it can be said that humans have a weakness for such foods.

• It is difficult to get rid of habits that have been ingrained in certain cultures. We have been raised with meat consumption for a long time, so trying to get rid of the habit is not an easy task.

• There is something that you need to know about the human body: it is truly adaptable. Because of our long-term dependency on animal products, our bodies have grown accustomed to absorbing the proteins from the meat. Thus, it is not easy to prove that meat is harmful for us. We are already used to it!

• Many nutritional studies are confusing and do not present a clear picture on why plant-based diets are important. It does not help with the fact that when people are planning to shift to a plant-based diet, they end up with a list of rationales that don't do a good job of justifying the shift.

So, how can you cut back on meat? Here are five ways to do it.

• Have a meatless day so that you can get used to the idea of eating plant-based food. Once you get used to having one meatless day in a week, increase it to two. Keep on doing it to other days until you have fully ingrained a meatless diet into your life. One of the best ways to do it is to do it during the weekends so that you have enough time to prepare some of the recipes from this book.

• During those meatless days, make sure that you are preparing some delicious plant-based food. Most people think that plant-based diets consist of bland foods that feature all the greens tossed in and blended together. While the blender does make its appearance in many recipes, plant-based food is not all about simply combining different natural ingredients. You do not have to sacrifice flavor for a new lifestyle.

• Here is another trick that you can adopt to curb your meat consumption. You can cut back on one meat product at a time. For example, you are quite used to having steak, bacon, and fish. Instead of simply stopping yourself from consuming all three items, start by removing the steak from your diet. Once you get used to its absence, work on getting rid of the next product. Keep on moving up the line until you have removed all the meaty ingredients from your life.

• Modify your favorite recipes and turn them into a complete plant-based meal. This might not be possible with all dishes, but look for ways you can change the recipe of some meals you enjoy immensely. For example, if you have been having beef Bolognese, then you can start off by replacing the recipe with one for vegetarian version of it. This will allow you to keep most of the flavors but add in a healthy twist. This is particularly useful when you have cravings for a certain dish. You may not be willing to easily let go of those cravings. But by discovering a delicious and healthier alternative, you might just be compelled to give up on the meat dish!

• You can even try to have one plant-based meal a day. Once you get used to the idea, you can extend it to two meals a day.

Vegan vs. Plant-Based Diet: Is There a Difference?

The two terms might sound like they can be interchanged. However, that is where people are usually mistaken. There are quite a few differences between a whole-food, plant-based diet and a vegan diet. Let us take a look at the table below.

Food/Inclusions	Vegan Diet	Whole-Food, Plant-Based Diet
Meat and Poultry	Not included	Not included
Seafood	Not included	Not included
Eggs and Dairy Products	Not included	Not included
Oils	Included	Not included
Highly Processed Foods	Included	Not included
Whole Grains	Included	Included
Fruits, Vegetables	Included	Included

Nuts and Seeds	Included	Included
Legumes	Included	Included

As you can see from the table above, vegan diet comes with certain types of oils and highly-processed foods. The important thing to note here is that whole-food, plant-based diet is a complete health booster that focuses on wholesome meals that give you the nutrients that your body requires.

Chapter 9: Planning Your Pantry

Usually, you do not have to worry about stocking up on food for your plant-based lifestyle. You can find all you need at the local grocery store or market. If you are choosing to store your food, then I would recommend getting transparent jars. This makes it easy to identify your ingredients and makes your pantry look colorful as well (nothing like products of nature to liven up your pantry). If you prefer to have the space for it, you can think about dedicating shelves for different purposes. For example, you can have an entire shelf for various spices, fruits, nuts, and seeds. The option is entirely up to you. Make sure you arrange your pantry in a way that is convenient to you. Here are some additional tips you can follow as a quick food guide for your pantry.

• Add in some flavor. You do not have to miss out on some healthy condiments. You can choose from options such as salsa, pesto, tahini, hummus, guacamole, and sauerkraut, to name a few.

• When you want a few replacements for white flour, you can always get quinoa or teff flour.

• Stock up on whole-grain foods whenever you notice a sale at your local store. This way, you end up saving more, and you do not have to spend on individual products.

• Always make sure that you have your basic baking items with you. Apart from choosing the right kind of flour, you should ideally have baking soda and baking powder (yes, both are necessary).

Pantry Stocking Tips

1. Protect your whole grains from bugs or mold The best way to go about this is by locking them in airtight containers. You should also keep them in a cool and dry place. One trick that I would recommend is putting labels on the containers that tell you the date of purchase of the grain. This helps you plan your meals better and avoid the situation where you pick the container up, open the lid, smell the contents, and wonder whether it is good to go or smells like it is home to some sort of microbe invasion.

2. Stock up on canned beans because they add more content to the food you are preparing However, make sure that you are not picking any beans that are high in sodium or salt. The labels will help you decide on what you are looking for. Make sure that you are aware of the other ingredients as well.

3. If you love cereals, then don't remove them entirely You don't have to be a cereal killer! Simply pick the ones that are low on sugar and have whole-grain ingredients. That way, you get to enjoy your breakfast (although there are some lip-smacking recipes that might just make you forget). What about oats, you say? You can find whole-grain and gluten-free oats in the market

that will fit your purposes. In fact, one can say that they are pretty outlandish!

4. Throw in a couple of your favorite hot sauces as well if you like to heat things up a bit A little spice is not going to bite. Or maybe it does.

Chapter 10: Breakfast

Fruity Granola

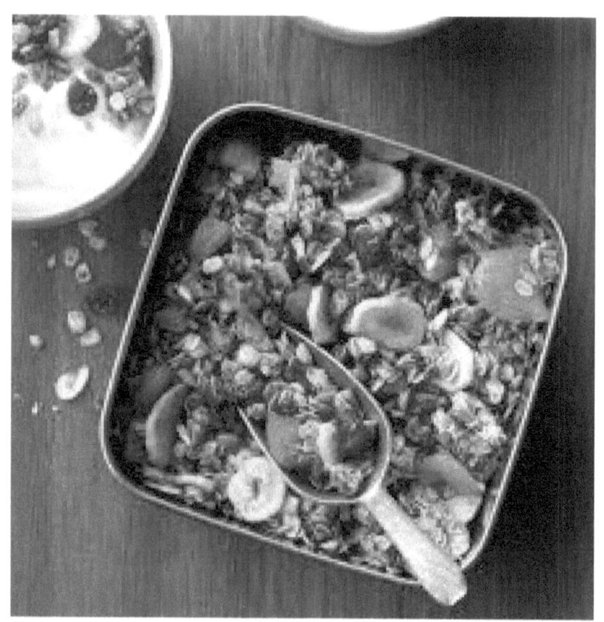

Preparation time: 50 minutes

Cooking time: 30 minutes

Servings: 4

Ingredients

2 cups rolled oats

¾ cup whole-grain flour

1 tablespoon ground cinnamon

1 teaspoon ground ginger (optional)

½ cup sunflower seeds, or walnuts, chopped

½ cup almonds, chopped

½ cup pumpkin seeds

½ cup unsweetened shredded coconut

1¼ cups pure fruit juice (cranberry, apple, or something similar)

½ cup raisins, or dried cranberries

½ cup goji berries (optional)

Directions

Preparing the Ingredients.

Preheat the oven to 350°F.

Mix together the oats, flour, cinnamon, ginger, sunflower seeds, almonds, pumpkin seeds, and coconut in a large bowl.

Sprinkle the juice over the mixture, and stir until it's just moistened. You might need a bit more or a bit less liquid, depending on how much your oats and flour absorb.

Spread the granola on a large baking sheet (the more spread out it is the better), and put it in the oven. After about 15 minutes, use a spatula to turn the granola so that the middle gets dried out. Let the granola bake until it's as crunchy as you want it, about 30 minutes more.

Take the granola out of the oven and stir in the raisins and goji berries (if using). Store leftovers in an airtight container for up to 2 weeks.

Serve with nondairy milk and fresh fruit, use as a topper for morning porridge or a smoothie bowl to add a bit of crunch, or make a granola parfait by layering with nondairy yogurt or puréed banana.

Pumpkin Steel-Cut Oats

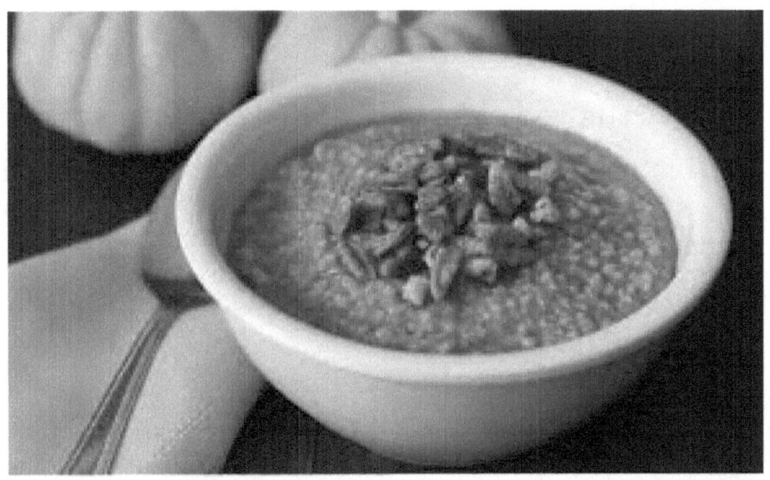

Preparation time: 5 minutes

Cooking time: 30 minutes

Servings: 4

Ingredients

3 cups water

1 cup steel-cut oats

½ cup canned pumpkin purée

¼ cup pumpkin seeds (pepitas)

2 tablespoons maple syrup

Pinch salt

Directions

Preparing the Ingredients.

In a large saucepan, bring the water to a boil.

Add the oats, stir, and reduce the heat to low. Simmer until the oats are soft, 20 to 30 minutes, continuing to stir occasionally.

Stir in the pumpkin purée and continue cooking on low for 3 to 5 minutes longer. Stir in the pumpkin seeds and maple syrup, and season with the salt.

Divide the oatmeal into 4 single-serving containers. Let cool before sealing the lids.

Place the containers in the refrigerator for up to 5 days.

Chocolate Quinoa Breakfast Bowl

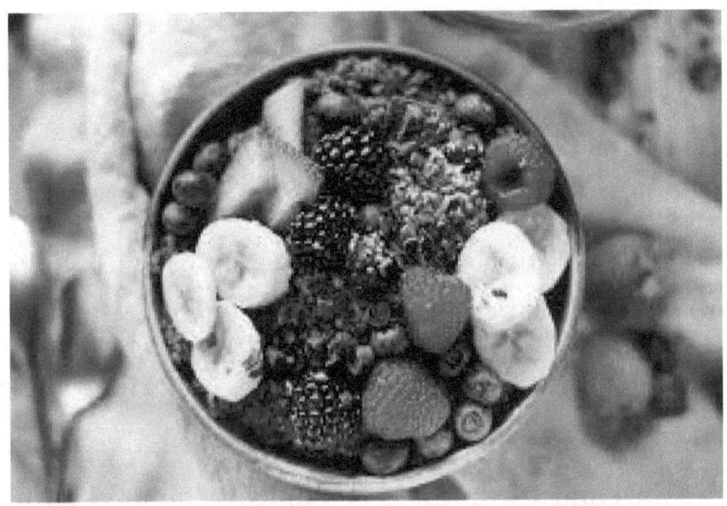

Preparation time: 10 minutes

Cooking time: 30 minutes

Servings: 4

Ingredients

1 cup quinoa

1 teaspoon ground cinnamon

1 cup nondairy milk

1 cup water

1 large banana

2 to 3 tablespoons unsweetened cocoa powder, or carob

1 to 2 tablespoons almond butter, or other nut or seed butter

1 tablespoon ground flaxseed, or chia or hemp seeds

2 tablespoons walnuts

¼ cup raspberries

Directions

Preparing the Ingredients.

Put the quinoa, cinnamon, milk, and water in a medium pot. Bring to a boil over high heat, then turn down low and simmer, covered, for 25 to 30 minutes.

While the quinoa is simmering, purée or mash the banana in a medium bowl and stir in the cocoa powder, almond butter, and flaxseed.

To serve, spoon 1 cup cooked quinoa into a bowl, top with half the pudding and half the walnuts and raspberries.

Savory Oatmeal Porridge

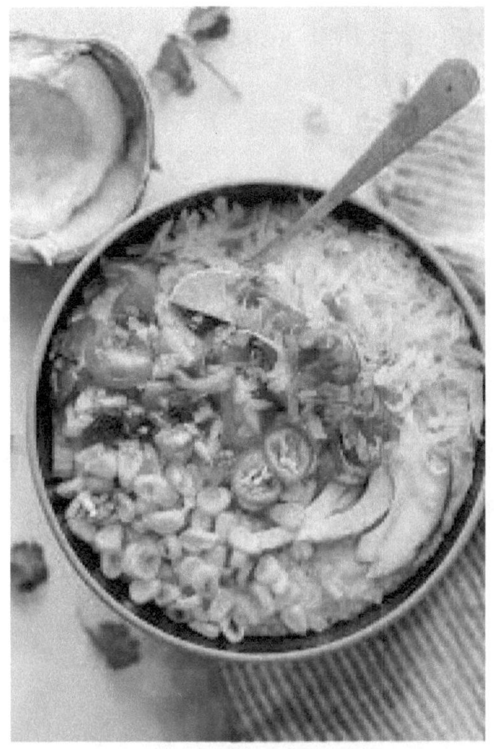

Preparation time: 10 mi nutes Cooking time: 40 minutes

Servings: 4

Ingredients

2½ cups vegetable broth

2½ cups unsweetened almond milk or other plant-based milk

½ cup steel-cut oats

1 tablespoon farro

½ cup slivered almonds

¼ cup nutritional yeast

2 cups old-fashioned rolled oats

½ teaspoon salt (optional)

Directions

Preparing the Ingredients.

In a large saucepan or pot, bring the broth and almond milk to a boil. Add the oats, farro, almond slivers, and nutritional yeast. Cook over medium-high heat for 20 minutes, stirring occasionally.

Add the rolled oats and cook for another 5 minutes, until creamy. Stir in the salt (if using).

Divide into 4 single-serving containers.

Let cool before sealing the lids. Place the containers in the refrigerator for up to 5 days.

Muesli and Berries Bowl

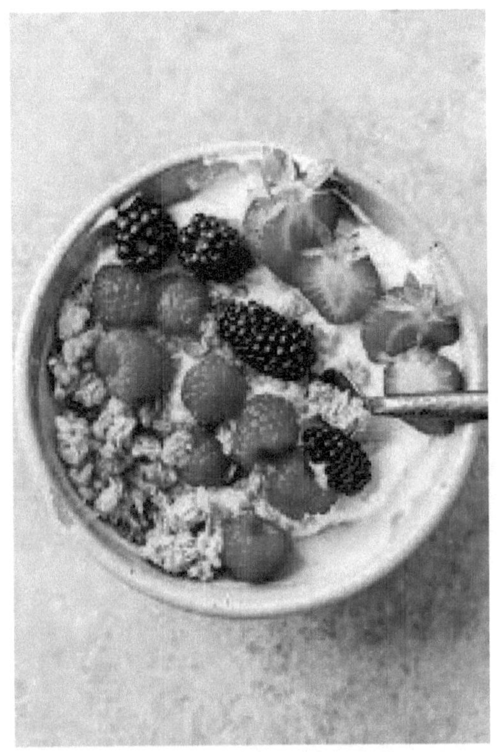

Preparation time: 10 minutes

Cooking time: 50 minutes

Servings: 4

Ingredients

FOR THE MUESLI

1 cup rolled oats

1 cup spelt flakes, or quin oa flakes, or more rolled oats

2 cups puffed cereal

¼ cup sunflower seeds

¼ cup almonds

¼ cup raisins

¼ cup dried cranberries

¼ cup chopped dried figs

¼ cup unsweetened shredded coconut

¼ cup nondairy chocolate chips

1 to 3 teaspoons ground cinnamon

FOR THE BOWL

½ cup nondairy milk, or unsweetened applesauce

¾ cup muesli

½ cup berries

Directions

Preparing the Ingredients.

Put the muesli ingredients in a container or bag and shake.

Combine the muesli and bowl ingredients in a bowl or to-go container.

Substitutions: Try chopped Brazil nuts, peanuts, dried cranberries, dried blueberries, dried mango, or whatever inspires you. Ginger and cardamom are interesting flavors if you want to branch out on spices.

Cinnamon And Spice Overnight Oats

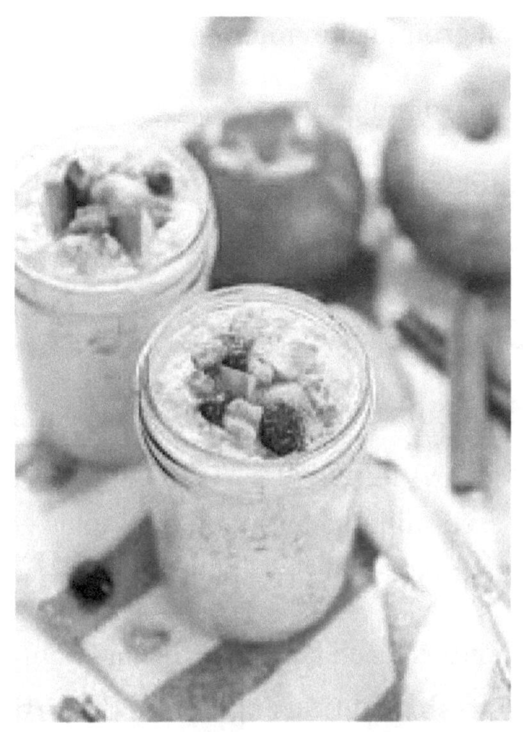

Preparation time: 5 minutes

Cooking time: 30 minutes

Servings: 4

Ingredients

2½ cups old-fashioned rolled oats

5 tablespoons pumpkin seeds (pepitas)

5 tablespoons chopped pecans

5 cups unsweetened plant-based milk

2½ teaspoons maple syrup or agave syrup

½ to 1 teaspoon salt

½ to 1 teaspoon ground cinnamon

½ to 1 teaspoon ground ginger

Fresh fruit (optional)

Directions

Preparing the Ingredients.

Line up 5 wide-mouth pint jars. In each jar, combine ½ cup of oats, 1 tablespoon of pumpkin seeds, 1 tablespoon of pecans, 1 cup of plant-based milk, ½ teaspoon of maple syrup, 1 pinch of salt, 1 pinch of cinnamon, and 1 pinch of ginger.

Stir the ingredients in each jar. Close the jars tightly with lids. To serve, top with fresh fruit (if using). Place the airtight jars in the refrigerator at least overnight before eating and for up to 5 days.

Baked Banana French Toast with Raspberry Syrup

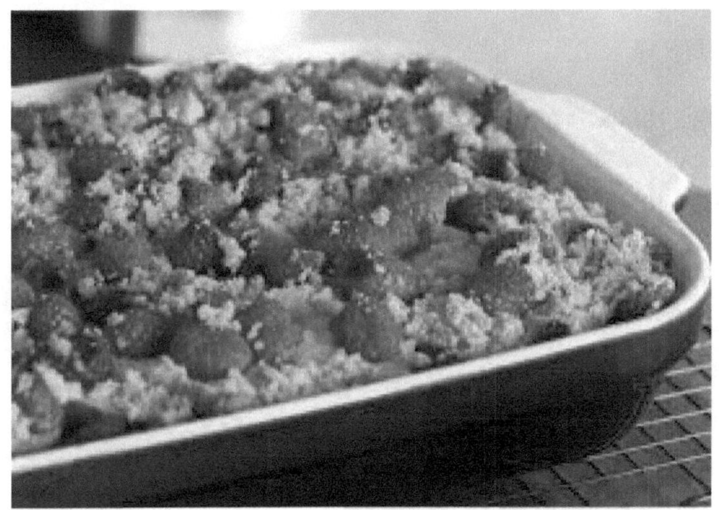

Preparation time: 10 minutes

Cooking time: 35 minutes

Servings: 4

Ingredients

FOR THE FRENCH TOAST

1 banana

1 cup coconut milk

1 teaspoon pure vanilla extract

¼ teaspoon ground nutmeg

½ teaspoon ground cinnamon

1½ teaspoons arrowroot powder

Pinch sea salt

8 slices whole-grain bread

FOR THE RASPBERRY SYRUP

1 cup fresh or frozen raspberries, or other berries

2 tablespoons water, or pure fruit juice

1 to 2 tablespoons maple syrup, or coconut sugar (optional)

Directions

Preparing the Ingredients.

Preheat the oven to 350°F.

In a shallow bowl, purée or mash the banana well. Mix in the coconut milk, vanilla, nutmeg, cinnamon, arrowroot, and salt.

Dip the slices of bread in the banana mixture, and then lay them out in a 13-by-9-inch baking dish. They should cover the bottom of the dish and can overlap a bit but shouldn't be stacked on top of each other. Pour any leftover banana mixture over the bread, and put the dish in the oven.

Bake about 30 minutes, or until the tops are lightly browned.

Serve topped with raspberry syrup.

To Make the Raspberry Syrup

Heat the raspberries in a small pot with the water and the maple syrup (if using) on medium heat.

Leave to simmer, stirring occasionally and breaking up the berries, for 15 to 20 minutes, until the liquid has reduced.

Leftover raspberry syrup makes a great topping for simple oatmeal as a quick and delicious breakfast, or as a drizzle on top of whole-grain toast smeared with natural peanut butter.

Great Green Smoothie

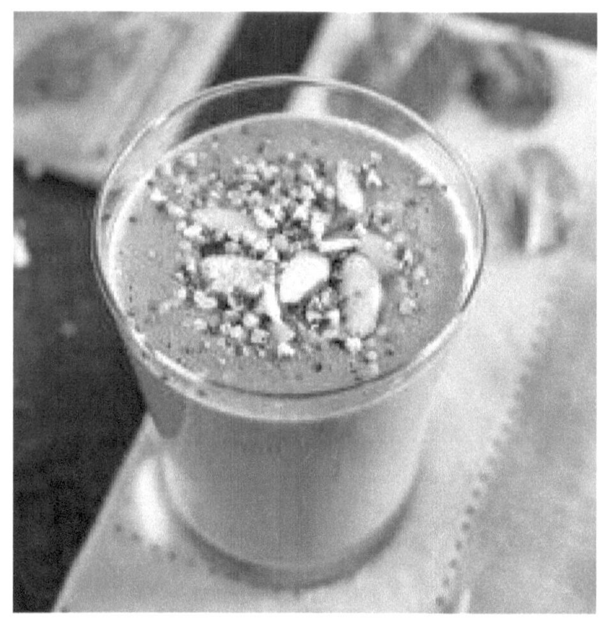

Preparation time: 10 minutes

Servings: 4

Ingredients

4 bananas, peeled

4 cups hulled strawberries

4 cups spinach

4 cups plant-based milk

Directions

Preparing the Ingredients.

Open 4 quart-size, freezer-safe bags. In each, layer in the following order: 1 banana (halved or sliced), 1 cup of strawberries, and 1 cup of spinach. Seal and place in the freezer.

To serve, take a frozen bag of Great Green Smoothie ingredients and transfer to a blender. Add 1 cup of plant-based milk, and blend until smooth. Place freezer bags in the freezer for up to 2 months.

Sunshine Muffins

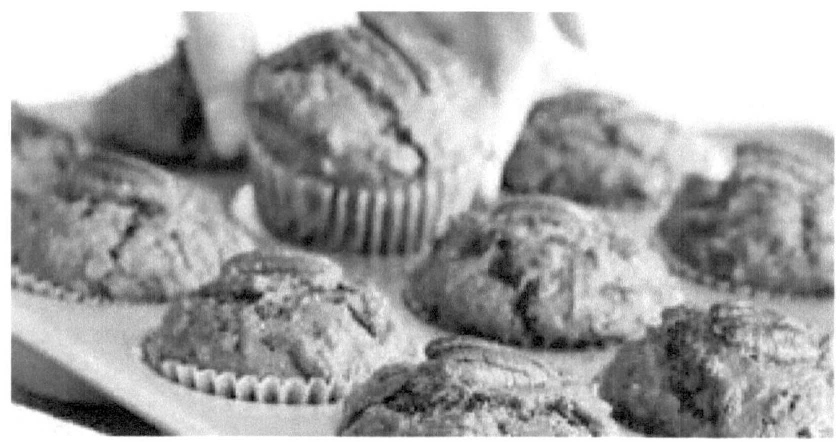

Preparation time: 10 minutes

Cooking time: 30 minutes

Servings: 4

Ingredients

1 teaspoon coconut oil, for greasing muffin tins (optional)

2 tablespoons almond butter, or sunflower seed butter

¼ cup nondairy milk

1 orange, peeled

1 carrot, coarsely chopped

2 tablespoons chopped dried apricots, or other dried fruit

3 tablespoons molasses

2 tablespoons ground flaxseed

1 teaspoon apple cider vinegar

1 teaspoon pure vanilla extract

½ teaspoon ground cinnamon

½ teaspoon ground ginger (optional)

¼ teaspoon ground nutmeg (optional)

¼ teaspoon allspice (optional)

¾ cup rolled oats, or whole-grain flour

1 teaspoon baking powder

½ teaspoon baking soda

MIX-INS (OPTIONAL)

½ cup rolled oats

2 tablespoons raisins, or other chopped dried fruit

2 tablespoons sunflower seeds

Directions

Preparing the Ingredients.

Preheat the oven to 350°F.

Prepare a 6-cup muffin tin by rubbing the insides of the cups with coconut oil or using silicone or paper muffin cups.

Purée the nut butter, milk, orange, carrot, apricots, molasses, flaxseed, vinegar, vanilla, cinnamon, ginger, nutmeg, and allspice in a food processor or blender until somewhat smooth.

Grind the oats in a clean coffee grinder until they're the consistency of flour (or use whole-grain flour). In a large bowl, mix the oats with the baking powder and baking soda. Mix the wet ingredients into the dry ingredients until just combined. Fold in the mix-ins (if using). Spoon about ¼ cup batter into each muffin cup and bake for 30 minutes, or until a toothpick inserted into the center comes out clean.

The orange creates a very moist base, so the muffins may take longer than 30 minutes, depending on how heavy your muffin tin is. Store the muffins in the fridge or freezer, because they are so moist. If you plan to keep them frozen, you can easily double the batch for a full dozen.

Smoothie Breakfast Bowl

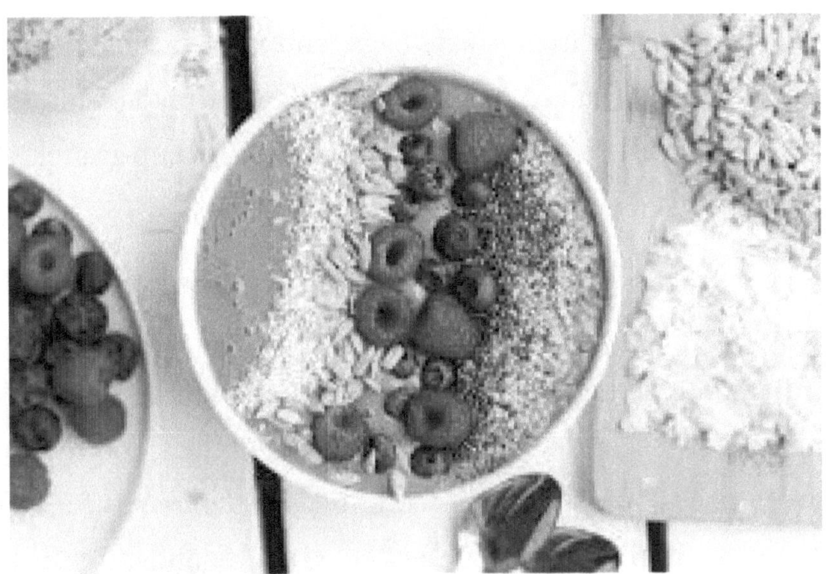

Preparation time: 10 minutes

Servings: 4

Ingredients

4 bananas, peeled

1 cup dragon fruit or fruit of choice

1 cup Baked Granola

2 cups fresh berries

½ cup slivered almonds

4 cups plant-based milk

Directions

Preparing the Ingredients.

Open 4 quart-size, freezer-safe bags, and layer in the following order: 1 banana (halved or sliced) and ¼ cup dragon fruit. Into 4 small jelly jars, layer in the following order: ¼ cup granola, ½ cup berries, and 2 tablespoons slivered almonds.

To serve, take a frozen bag of bananas and dragon fruit and transfer to a blender. Add 1 cup of plant-based milk, and blend until smooth. Pour into a bowl. Add the contents of 1 jar of granola, berries, and almonds over the top of the smoothie, and serve with a spoon. Place the freezer bags in the freezer for up to 2 months. Store the jars of berries, granola, and nuts in the refrigerator for up to 1 week.

Pink Panther Smoothie

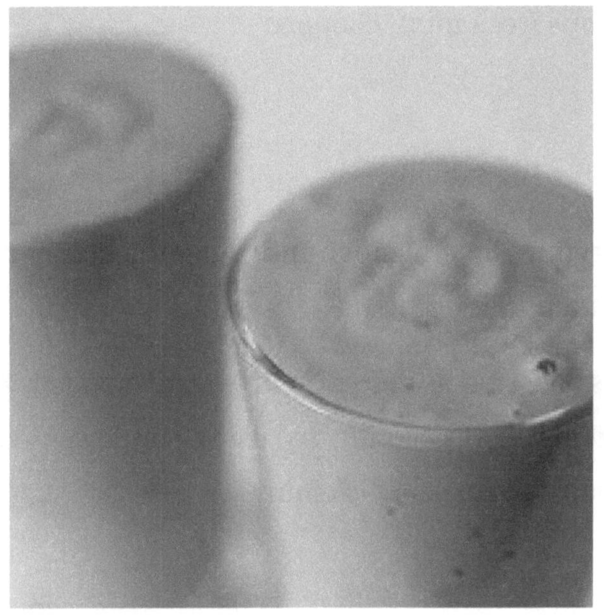

Preparation time: 10 minutes

Servings: 4

Ingredients

1 cup strawberries

1 cup chopped melon (any kind)

1 cup cranberries, or raspberries

1 tablespoon chia seeds

½ cup coconut milk, or other nondairy milk

1 cup water

(OPTIONAL)

1 teaspoon goji berries

2 tablespoons fresh mint, chopped

Directions

Preparing the Ingredients.

Purée everything in a blender until smooth, adding more water (or coconut milk) if needed.

Add bonus boosters, as desired. Purée until blended. If you don't have (or don't like) coconut, try using sunflower seeds for an immune boost of zinc and selenium.

Tortilla Breakfast Casserole

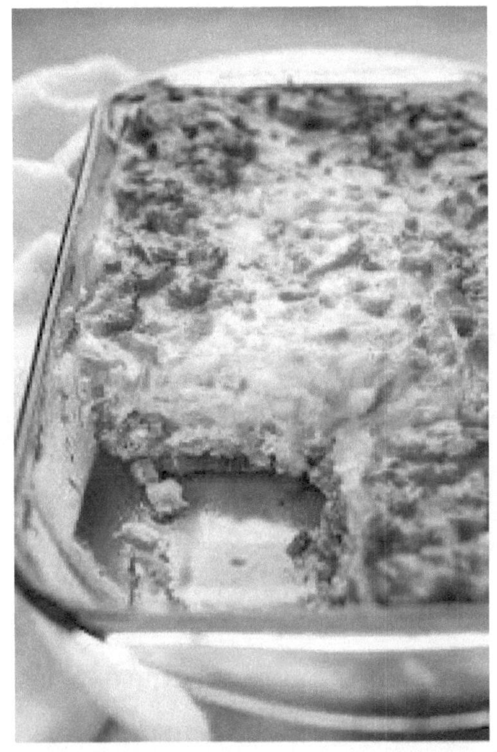

Preparation time: 10 minutes

Cooking time: 30 minutes

Servings: 4

Ingredients

Nonstick cooking spray

1 recipe Tofu-Spinach Scramble

1 (14-ounce) can black beans, rinsed and drained

¼ cup nutritional yeast

2 teaspoons hot sauce

10 small corn tortillas

½ cup shredded vegan Cheddar or pepper Jack cheese, divided

Directions

Preparing the Ingredients.

Preheat the oven to 350°F.

Coat a 9-by-9-inch baking pan with cooking spray.

In a large bowl, combine the tofu scramble with the black beans, nutritional yeast, and hot sauce. Set aside.

In the bottom of the baking pan, place 5 corn tortillas. Spread half of the tofu and bean mixture over the tortillas. Spread ¼ cup of cheese over the top. Layer the remaining 5 tortillas over the top of the cheese. Spread the reminder of the tofu and bean mixture over the tortillas. Spread the remaining ¼ cup of cheese over the top.

Bake for 20 minutes. Divide evenly among 6 single-serving containers. Let cool before sealing the lids. Place the containers in the refrigerator for up to 5 days.

If you want to keep the casserole intact in the freezer, consider baking it in a disposable pan. Once cool, simply cover with foil and freeze.

Tofu-Spinach Scramble

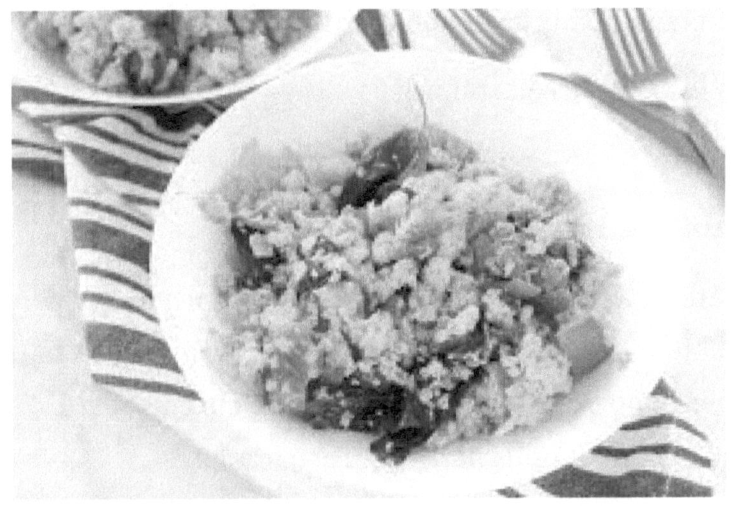

Preparation time: 10 minutes

Cooking time: 40 minutes

Servings: 4

Ingredients

1 (14-ounce) package water-packed extra-firm tofu

1 teaspoon extra-virgin olive oil or ¼ cup vegetable broth

1 small yellow onion, diced

3 teaspoons minced garlic (about 3 cloves)

3 large celery stalks, chopped

2 large carrots, peeled (optional) and chopped

1 teaspoon chili powder

½ teaspoon ground cumin

½ teaspoon ground turmeric

½ teaspoon salt (optional)

¼ teaspoon freshly ground black pepper

5 cups loosely packed spinach

Directions

Preparing the Ingredients.

Press and drain the tofu by placing it, wrapped in a paper towel, on a plate in the sink. Place a cutting board over the tofu, then set a heavy pot, can, or cookbook on the cutting board. Remove after 10 minutes. (Alternatively, use a tofu press.)

In a medium bowl, crumble the tofu with your hands or a potato masher. Set aside.

In a large skillet over medium-high heat, heat the olive oil. Add the onion, garlic, celery, and carrots, and sauté for 5 minutes, until the onion is softened.

Add the crumbled tofu, chili powder, cumin, turmeric, salt (if using), and pepper, and continue cooking for 7 to 8 more minutes, stirring frequently, until the tofu begins to brown.

Add the spinach and mix well. Cover and reduce the heat to medium. Steam the spinach for 3 minutes.

Divide evenly among 5 single-serving containers. Let cool before sealing the lids.

Place the containers in the refrigerator for up to 5 days.

Mango Madness

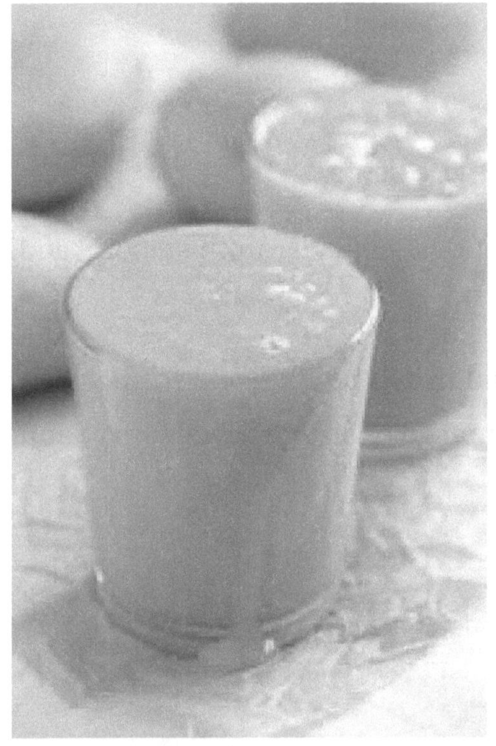

Preparation time: 10 minutes

Cooking time: 30 minutes

Servings: 4

Ingredients

1 banana

1 cup chopped mango (frozen or fresh)

1 cup chopped peach (frozen or fresh)

1 cup strawberries

1 carrot, peeled and chopped (optional)

1 cup water

Directions

Preparing the Ingredients.

Purée everything in a blender until smooth, adding more water
if needed.

If you can't find frozen peaches and fresh ones aren't in season,
just use extra mango or strawberries, or try cantaloupe.

Savory Pancakes

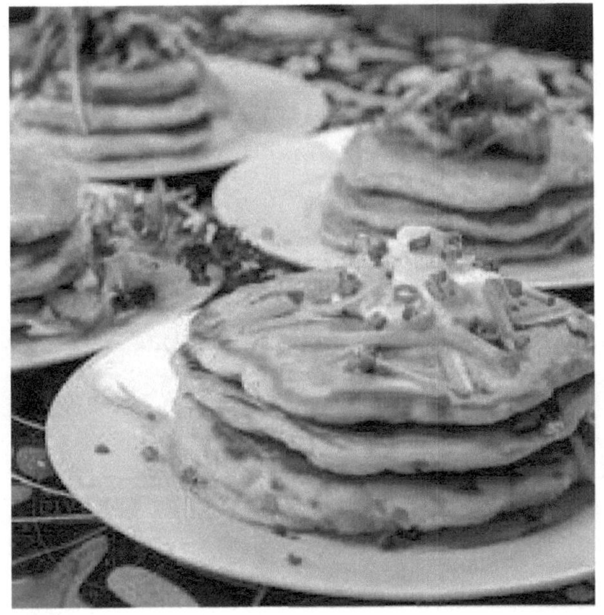

Preparation time: 10 minutes

Cooking time: 30 minutes

Servings: 4

Ingredients

1 cup whole-wheat flour

1 teaspoon garlic salt

1 teaspoon onion powder

½ teaspoon baking soda

¼ teaspoon salt

1 cup lightly pressed, crumbled soft or firm tofu

⅓ cup unsweetened plant-based milk

¼ cup lemon juice (about 2 small lemons)

2 tablespoons extra-virgin olive oil

½ cup finely chopped mushrooms

½ cup finely chopped onion

2 cups tightly packed greens (arugula, spinach, or baby kale work great)

Nonstick cooking spray

Directions

Preparing the Ingredients.

In a large bowl, combine the flour, garlic salt, onion powder, baking soda, and salt. Mix well. In a blender, combine the tofu, plant-based milk, lemon juice, and olive oil. Purée on high speed for 30 seconds.

Pour the contents of the blender into the bowl of dry ingredients and whisk until combined well. Fold in the mushrooms, onion, and greens.

Spray a large skillet or griddle pan with nonstick cooking spray and set over medium-high heat. Reduce the heat to medium and add ½ cup of batter per pancake. Cook on both sides for about 3 minutes, or until set. After flipping, press down on the cooked side of the pancake with a spatula to flatten out the pancake. Repeat until the batter is gone.

Divide the cooked pancakes among 4 single-serving containers. Let cool before sealing the lids.

Place the airtight storage containers in the refrigerator for up to 4 days. To reheat, microwave for 1½ to 2 minutes. To freeze, place the pancakes on a parchment paper–lined baking sheet in a single layer. If there's more than one layer, place another piece of parchment paper over the pancakes and place the second layer on top. Place the baking sheet in the freezer for 2 to 4 hours. Transfer the frozen pancakes to a freezer-safe bag (cut the parchment paper and place a small piece between each pancake). To thaw, refrigerate overnight. Preheat an oven or toaster oven to 350°F. Place the pancakes on a parchment paper–lined baking sheet and bake for 10 to 15 minutes, or stack the pancakes on a plate and microwave for 2 to 3 minutes.

Chapter 11: Lunch

Asian-Inspired Teriyaki Veggie Burgers with Shitake Mushrooms

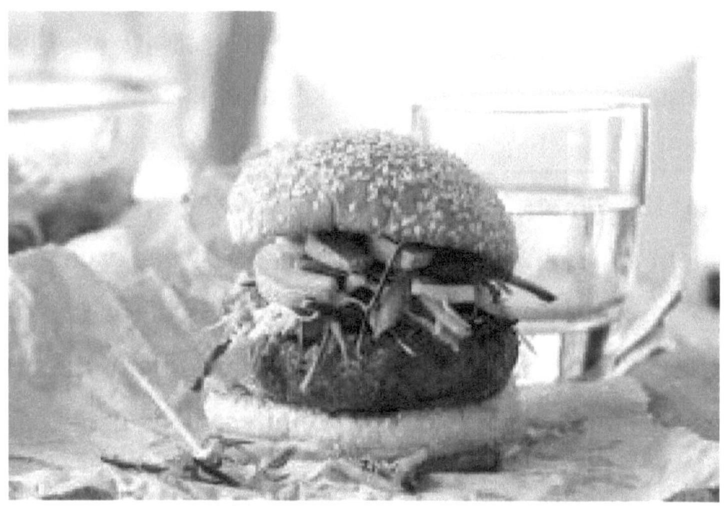

Preparation time: 10 minutes

Cooking time: 60 minutes

Servings: 4

Ingredients:

1 small sweet potato, about ½ pound

¾ cup old-fashioned rolled oats

1 15-ounce can kidney beans, rinsed and drained

2 green onions, thinly sliced

½ cup shelled sunflower seeds

½ teaspoon kosher salt

½ teaspoon garlic powder

2 teaspoons paprika

1¾ tablespoons mirin, divided

4 shiitake mushrooms, stems removed

1 tablespoon olive or coconut oil

2 teaspoons sriracha

¼ cup vegan mayonnaise

Whole wheat English muffins

Alfalfa sprouts

Directions:

Preheat the oven to 375 degrees, Fahrenheit.

Prick the sweet potato with a fork and heat on high in the microwave for about eight minutes. Turn the potato over and microwave it for eight more minutes or until cooked through. Cool and cut in half lengthwise.

Spread out the oats on a cutting board and chop them coarsely. Pour into a mixing bowl.

Rinse and drain the beans and place them in the bowl with the oats.

Chop the green onions and add them to the bowl.

Add the sunflower seeds, salt, garlic powder, paprika, 1½ tablespoons of the mirin and 1½ tablespoons of the soy sauce; mix everything together with your hands, mashing the beans.

Remove the skin from the cooked sweet potato and put it in the bowl as well. Mix everything together with your hands.

Shape four patties and set them on a rimmed baking sheet that has been covered with parchment paper. Bake for 15 minutes on one side, turn and cook for another 15 minutes on the other side. Cool for five minutes.

While the patties are cooking, slice the four mushroom caps and use the stems to make vegetable broth.

Set a skillet over medium heat, place in it the oil and let it warm up.

Add the remaining mirin and soy sauce to the skillet, then add the mushrooms and sauté for about a minute.

In a bowl, mix the sriracha with the mayonnaise.

Place the burgers on an English muffin with mushroom mixture on top and alfalfa sprouts on top of that. Put some of the sriracha mixture on the inside of the muffin top and use it to close the sandwich.

Barbeque Bean Tacos with Tropical Salsa

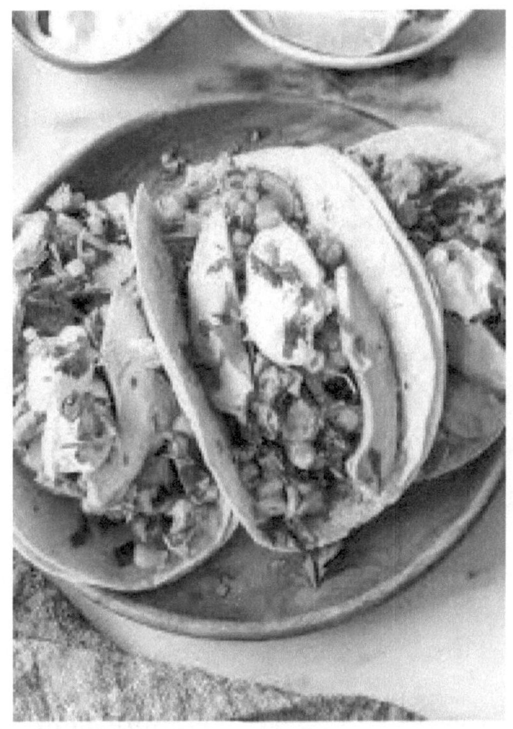

Preparation time: 10 minutes

Cooking time: 30 minutes

Servings: 4

Ingredients:

2 15-ounce cans pinto beans (substitution: white beans)

1 tablespoon maple syrup

2 tablespoons prepared Dijon mustard

½ teaspoon chili powder

½ teaspoon garlic powder

¾ teaspoon sea salt, divided

1 20-ounce can pineapple chunks, packed in juice

¼ cup cilantro, finely chopped (plus more for garnish)

¼ cup red onion, minced

3 radishes, stemmed and thinly sliced

1 small green cabbage, cored and thinly sliced

1 lime, cut into wedges

4 corn tortillas

Directions:

Drain and rinse the beans and pour into a heavy skillet.

Add the maple syrup, mustard, ketchup, chili powder, garlic powder and a half teaspoon of salt. Heat on low, stirring frequently, until the mixture heats through and thickens.

Meanwhile, drain and chop the pineapple chunks and put them in a bowl.

Add the cilantro, onion and the remaining salt and stir together.

Take a tortilla and place a fourth of the bean mixture on the side. Sprinkle with the radish and cabbage mixture and top with the pineapple mixture. Garnish the tops with more cilantro. Serve with lime wedges.

Burgundy Mushroom Sauce Over Polenta

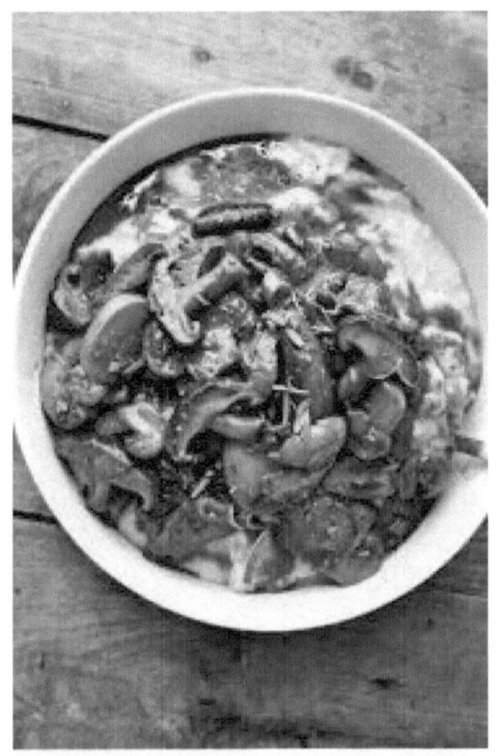

Preparation time: 10 minutes

Cooking time: 70 minutes

Servings: 4

Ingredients:

1 tablespoon olive oil

1 medium red onion, chopped

4 cloves garlic, minced

2 large carrots, peeled, cut in half and thinly sliced

24 ounces (3 8-ounce packages) Cremini mushrooms, sliced

1 teaspoon dry mustard

½ teaspoon dried rosemary

½ teaspoon dried thyme

½ teaspoon sea salt

½ teaspoon ground black pepper

1½ cups red wine

1 15-ounce can diced tomatoes

4 green onions, chopped

1 cup unsweetened nondairy milk or vegetable broth

¼ cup parsley, chopped

Directions:

In a large pot over medium heat, heat the olive oil and the onion. Sauté for two to three minutes.

Add the garlic, carrots, dry mustard, rosemary, thyme, salt and pepper and sauté until the mushrooms turn golden and lose most of their liquid.

Deglaze with the wine; scrape the brown bits up from the bottom of the pan.

Add the tomatoes, Worcestershire sauce and green onions. Cook to reduce the liquid by half.

Make some polenta, rice, or quinoa and set it aside until ready to serve.

If you're using polenta, stir in enough of the nondairy milk or vegetable broth until it becomes the consistency of mashed potatoes.

To serve, spoon the mushroom sauce over the polenta and sprinkle with the parsley.

Carrot Brown Rice Casserole With Spinach

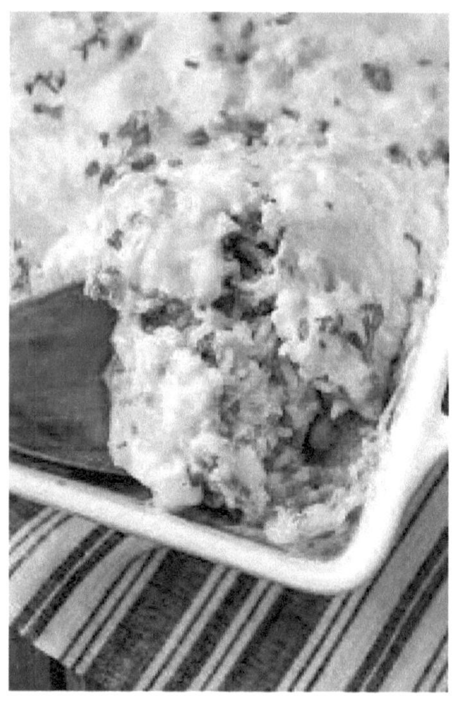

Preparation time: 10 minutes

Cooking time: 30 minutes

Servings: 4

Ingredients:

1 bunch fresh spinach leaves, chopped

3 cups shredded carrots

1 large onion, chopped

1 teaspoon sea salt

½ teaspoon dry thyme

1½ teaspoons garlic powder

3 cups water or vegetable stock

3 cups cooked brown rice

¾ cup whole-grain crumbs

Directions:

Coat the inside of a two-quart casserole with nonstick spray and preheat the oven to 350 degrees, Fahrenheit.

Spread the spinach on the bottom of the casserole dish.

Heat a large pot over medium high heat and add the two tablespoons of vegetable broth. This will keep everything from sticking to the pan.

Add the onions and carrots and sauté for five minutes.

Add the salt, thyme and garlic powder and stir in.

Add the peanut butter and water or vegetable stock and whisk until smooth.

Stir in the soy sauce along with the breadcrumbs and stir well.

Pour this on top of the spinach and cover with a lid or foil.

Bake for 45 minutes and take out of the oven. Let cool for 10 minutes, remove the cover and serve.

Cashew Topped Vegetable Stuffed Peppers

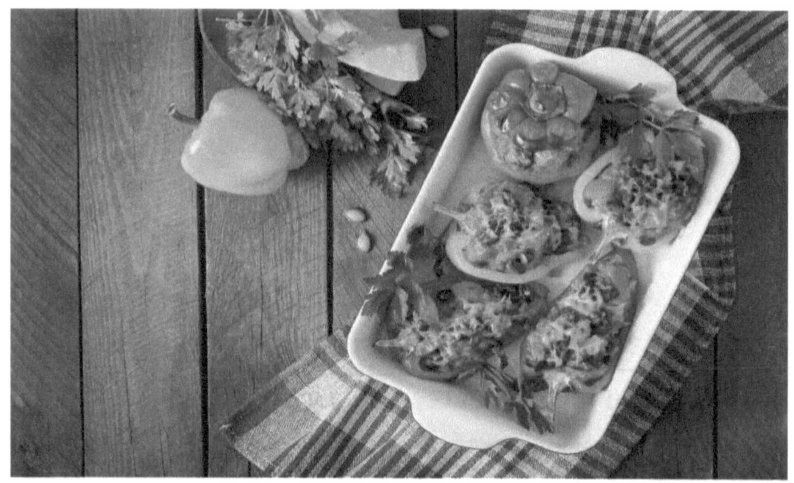

Preparation time: 10 minutes

Cooking time: 30 minutes

Servings: 4

Ingredients:

1 tablespoon olive oil

2 cloves garlic, chopped

1 medium onion, chopped

8 ounces mushrooms, sliced

2 to three large Swiss chard leaves, coarsely chopped

1 15-ounce can kidney beans, rinsed and drained

8 sun-dried tomatoes, soaked in hot water until reconstituted and chopped

1 to 2 cups tomato sauce

1½ cups cooked brown rice or quinoa

3 large red peppers, cut into half lengthwise

⅓ cup raw cashews, finely chopped

Directions:

Preheat the oven to 375 degrees, Fahrenheit.

Place the olive oil in a heated skillet and add the garlic, sautéing for two minutes.

Add the onions and mushrooms and sauté until the onion is soft.

Add the chard and beans and cook until the chard wilts.

Add the drained and chopped sun-dried tomatoes, tomato sauce and cooked rice or quinoa. Stir to combine everything.

Fill the pepper cups with the mixture and place in a baking dish that has been sprayed with nonstick spray. Cover with foil.

Bake for 40 minutes, remove from the oven and sprinkle cashews over the top. Bake for another 10 minutes.

Cool for 10 minutes before serving.

Coconut Curry With Cauliflower and Tomato

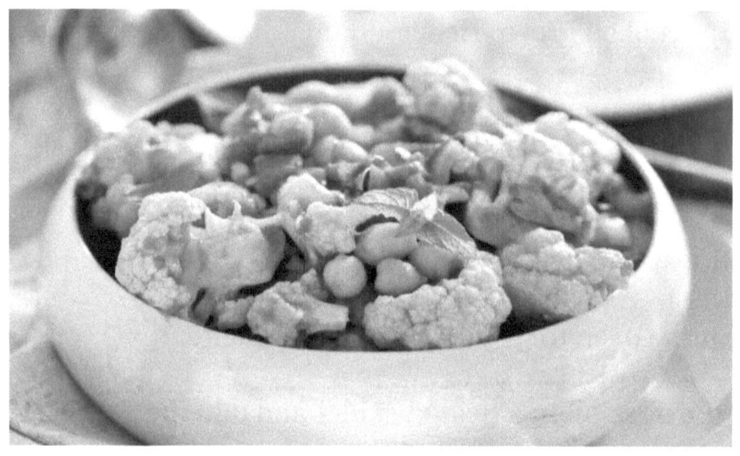

Preparation time: 10 minutes

Cooking time: 50 minutes

Servings: 4

Ingredients:

Cooked brown rice for serving

2 tablespoons olive oil

1 onion, chopped

1 pound (about 4 cups) sweet potato, unpeeled but chopped

1 head cauliflower (about 4 cups), chopped

1 teaspoon kosher salt, divided

1 tablespoon garam masala

1 teaspoon cumin

¼ teaspoon cayenne pepper

2 tablespoons curry powder

1 23-ounce jar diced San Marzano plum tomatoes

1 15-ounce can full-fat coconut milk

1 15-ounce can chickpeas, rinsed and drained

4 cups fresh spinach leaves

Cilantro for garnish

Directions:

Heat the oil in a large pot over medium heat.

Sauté the onions for about three minutes, then add the sweet potato and sauté for another 3 minutes.

Add the cauliflower and a half teaspoon of the salt; sauté for five minutes.

Add the garam marsala, cumin, cayenne pepper and curry powder; stir to mix thoroughly.

Pour in the plum tomatoes, including their juice and the coconut milk; bring to a boil.

Reduce the heat and simmer, covered, for about 10 minutes. The cauliflower should be soft.

Add the chickpeas and spinach leaves, along with the rest of the salt; stir until the spinach wilts and the chickpeas are heated through.

Serve over brown rice and garnish with cilantro.

Greek Style Stuffed Sweet Potatoes

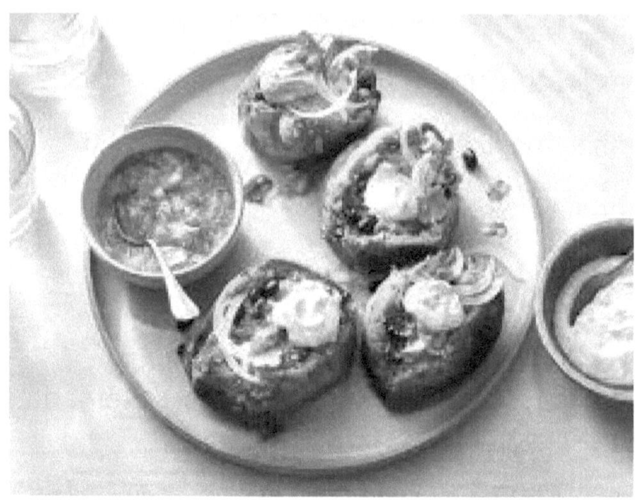

Preparation time: 10 minutes

Cooking time: 50 minutes

Servings: 4

Ingredients:

4 sweet potatoes

½ red onion, chopped

1 cucumber, peeled and chopped

2 large tomatoes, chopped

1 small jar Kalamata olives, chopped

3 tablespoons fresh mint, chopped

1 lime, juiced

1 clove garlic, processed into a paste

2 tablespoons lemon juice

⅓ cup Tahini sauce

¼ teaspoon salt

2 to 6 tablespoons lukewarm water

1 15-ounce can chickpeas, drained and rinsed

Directions:

Preheat the oven to 375 degrees, Fahrenheit.

Cut the cleaned sweet potatoes in half lengthwise and place them, with cut side down, on a greased baking sheet. Bake for 20 to 30 minutes, until tender when poked with a fork. Remove from the oven to cool.

In a bowl, combine the onions, cucumber, tomatoes, olives, mint and lime juice. Mix well and set the bowl aside.

In another bowl, combine the garlic, lemon juice, Tahini sauce and salt. Start adding the water with two tablespoons and see if it becomes the right consistency. If it is thick and pasty, add more of the water up to six tablespoons. Set the mixture aside.

To assemble, place two potato halves on a plate right side up and mash with a fork lightly. Place the onion, cucumber tomato and olive mixture on top. Sprinkle with chickpeas and end up with the Tahini mixture on top and serve.

Imitation Crab Cakes With Tofu

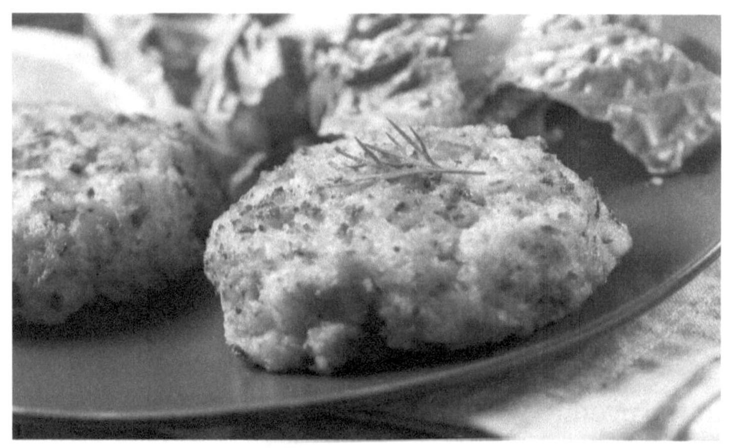

Preparation time: 10 minutes

Cooking time: 30 minutes

Servings: 4

Ingredients:

2 tablespoons ground flaxseed

4 tablespoons water

1 block tofu

½ cup red bell pepper, diced

½ cup yellow bell pepper, diced

¾ cup red onion, diced

1½ cups celery diced

¼ cup flat leaf parsley, chopped

1 tablespoons capers, drained

salt and pepper to taste

1 tablespoon lemon juice

½ tablespoon lemon zest

½ cup dry wheat bread crumbs

2 tablespoons Dijon mustard

Mango salsa, for accompaniment

Directions:

Combine the flaxseed and water and let it soak until ready to use.

Cut the tofu block in half lengthwise, pressing each half between paper towels and wrapping in newspaper to make it as dry as possible. Place something heavy on top and let it rest for 20 minutes.

Put the red and yellow bell pepper, the onion, celery, parsley, capers, Worcestershire sauce, hot sauce, Old Bay seasoning, vegetable stock, salt and pepper in a large pot over medium low heat. Cook for 15 minutes or until everything is soft. Cool to room temperature.

Place the tofu in a large bowl and mash it into small pieces

Add the lemon juice, lemon zest, breadcrumbs, mustard and the flaxseed, including the water. Mix well.

Add the vegetable mixture and mix well.

Cover the bowl and let it rest in the refrigerator for 30 minutes.

Preheat the oven to 375 degrees, Fahrenheit and cover a baking sheet with parchment paper.

Remove the mixture from the refrigerator and shape it into balls, place them on the parchment paper and press down to flatten.

Bake for five minutes on each side and serve with mango salsa.

Lentil and Mushroom Loaf (Fake Meatloaf)

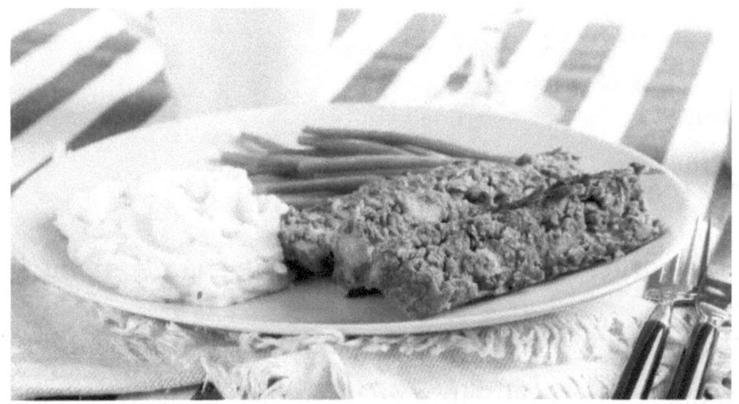

Preparation time: 10 minutes

Cooking time: 60 minutes

Servings: 4

Ingredients:

2 cloves garlic, finely chopped

1 small onion, chopped

3 cups mushrooms, finely chopped

1 cup green lentils, already cooked

1 cup red lentils, already cooked

½ cup old-fashioned rolled oats

¼ cup ground flaxseed

2 tablespoons dried thyme

½ teaspoon salt

¼ teaspoon pepper

2 tablespoons to ½ cup water

Directions:

Preheat the oven to 370 degrees, Fahrenheit.

Place the garlic, onion and mushrooms in a large mixing bowl.

Add the green and red lentils, oats, flaxseed, Tamari, thyme, salt and pepper; mix well with your hands. The mixture may be a little crumbly.

Add water, a little bit at a time and up to a half cup as needed until the mixture starts to stick together like a regular meatloaf. Add two tablespoons first, then add by two-tablespoon increments until the loaf gains the proper texture.

Place a strip of parchment paper on the bottom of the pan that extends up both sides and out of the pan on the small sides. This creates a sling that you can grasp to pull out the loaf after it's cooked.

Pack the loaf mixture into the pan and bake for 50 to 60 minutes.

Remove from oven and cool for 15 minutes. Lift the loaf out of the pan and set it on a cutting board to slice Serve while warm.

Meatless Chick Nuggets

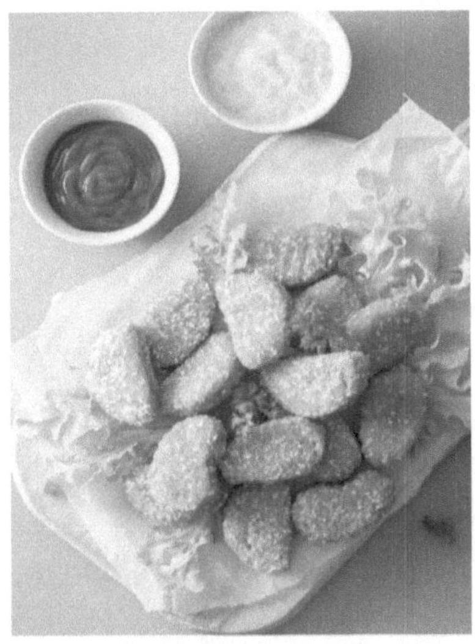

Preparation time: 10 minutes

Cooking time: 30 minutes

Servings: 4

Ingredients:

1 15.5-ounce can chickpeas, rinsed and drained

½ teaspoon garlic powder

1 teaspoon granulated onion

1 tablespoon nutritional yeast

1 tablespoon whole-wheat bread crumbs (optional: substitute panko bread crumbs)

½ cup panko bread crumbs

Directions:

Preheat the oven to 350 degrees, Fahrenheit and cover a rimmed baking pan with parchment paper.

Place the drained chickpeas in a food processor and pulse four to five times.

Add the garlic powder, granulated onion, nutritional yeast and the tablespoon of whole-wheat bread crumbs to the processor and process until you get a chunky, grainy mixture that sticks together.

Scoop out by teaspoonfuls and form balls.

Roll the balls in the panko crumbs and set on the baking sheet, flattening each ball so it looks more like a chicken nugget. Be sure to space them apart so they do not touch each other.

Bake for 20 minutes, remove from the oven and flip each nugget over with tongs. Return to the oven for 10 more minutes.

Cool for a few minutes and then serve with honey, barbecue sauce or Ranch dipping sauce.

Portobello Bolognese With Zucchini Noodles

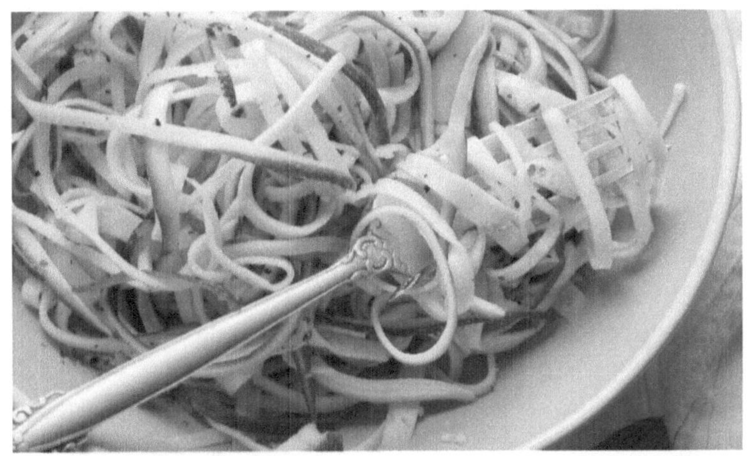

Preparation time: 10 minutes

Cooking time: 40 minutes

Servings: 4

Ingredients:

3 tablespoons olive oil, divided

½ cup onion, minced

3 cloves of garlic, minced

½ cup carrot, peeled and minced

½ cup celery, minced

6 portobello mushroom caps, stems removed and finely chopped

½ teaspoon Kosher salt

½ teaspoon ground pepper

1 28-ounce can crushed plum tomatoes

¼ teaspoon red pepper flakes, crushed (optional)

½ cup fresh basil leaves, finely chopped with more left whole for garnish

2 teaspoons dried oregano

4 medium zucchini

Directions:

Heat two tablespoons of the olive oil in a large skillet over medium high heat.

Add the onion, garlic, carrot and celery; sauté for about five minutes or until the onion turns translucent.

Add the mushrooms and sauté for another six to seven minutes, until the mushrooms shrink and lose their liquid. Stir constantly so they don't burn but turn a golden hue.

Stir in the tomato paste and cook, stirring frequently, for about two minutes.

Pour in the crushed tomatoes, red pepper flakes, basil and oregano. Reduce the heat to a simmer, cooking very low until the sauce thickens.

While the pot simmers, create the zucchini noodles and put them in cold water until they're all made. Drain the noodles and use tongs to place them in a skillet with a little water at the bottom. Toss and add some salt and pepper. They will only take a few minutes to soften and warm over medium heat.

Divide the noodles among four bowls and serve with the sauce on top; add a basil leaf on top as garnish.

Pot Roast Made with Portobello Mushrooms

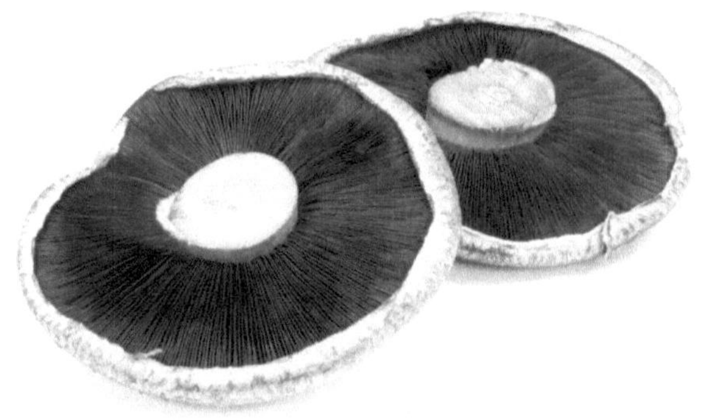

Preparation time: 10 minutes

Cooking time: 30 minutes

Servings: 4

Ingredients:

½ cup red wine, divided

4 large portobello mushroom caps, sliced into ¾-inch pieces

2 cloves garlic, smashed

1 large onion, sliced

1 teaspoon dried basil

1 teaspoon rubbed sage

3 tablespoons flour (I use white flour, but you can substitute whole grain flour)

½ teaspoon sea salt

½ teaspoon ground black pepper

4 large carrots, peeled and cut into thick pieces

4 large potatoes, peeled and cut into bite-sized pieces

1 sprig fresh rosemary

4 sprigs fresh thyme

Directions:

Preheat the oven to 350 degrees, Fahrenheit.

In a large saucepan, heat a quarter cup of wine with the portobello slices and let them cook down and brown, stirring frequently. Pour into a bowl and set aside.

Deglaze the pan the mushrooms were in, using the remaining red wine; add the garlic and onions. Sauté until the onions wilt and start to brown. Transfer to a different bowl and set it aside.

In a small bowl, whisk together the basil, sage and flour. Whisk in a quarter cup of the vegetable stock to make a sloppy paste and scrape all of it into the same saucepan you used for the mushrooms.

Stir constantly over medium heat and gradually add the remaining stock to create a gravy. Keep whisking to prevent lumps.

When the gravy starts to boil, turn off the heat and add the salt and pepper. If it seems too dry add a little extra stock and stir to combine.

Pour the mushroom mixture into the gravy and then add the onion mixture. Stir well.

Add the carrots, potatoes and Worcestershire sauce, stirring to combine.

Pour into a 2-quart glass casserole coated with nonstick spray. Top with the rosemary and thyme sprigs and cover with a lid or with foil.

Bake for one hour, then serve.

Quesadilla With Black Beans and Sweet Potato

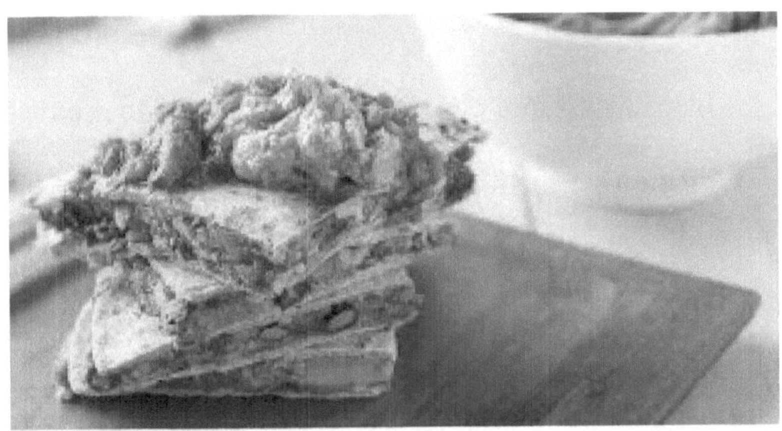

Preparation time: 10 minutes

Cooking time: 55 minutes

Servings: 4

Ingredients:

1 medium-sized sweet potato, peeled and cut into cubes

3 teaspoons taco seasoning

4 whole-wheat tortillas

½ of a 15-ounce can of black beans, drained and rinsed

Directions:

Bring a large pot of water to boil and drop in the sweet potato.

Boil for 10 to 20 minutes or until soft.

Drain the sweet potato and put in a bowl.

Add the taco seasoning and mash well.

To assemble the quesadilla, spread the sweet potato mixture on the tortilla.

Add the black beans and press them onto the potato mixture.

Cover with another tortilla.

Heat a nonstick skillet over medium high heat and lay the tortilla in it. Toast on both sides and serve immediately.

Quinoa-stuffed Acorn Squash

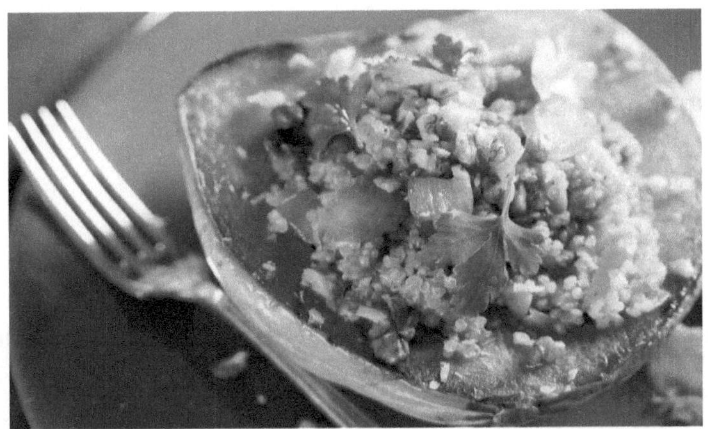

Preparation time: 10 minutes

Cooking time: 30 minutes

Servings: 4

Ingredients:

½ cup quinoa, cooked per package instructions

2 acorn squash

⅛ cup water

1 large onion, chopped

⅛ teaspoon ground cloves

⅛ teaspoon ground cardamom

½ teaspoon ground ginger

1 teaspoon ground cinnamon

½ cup raisins

⅓ cup walnuts or pecans, chopped

½ teaspoon sea salt

¼ teaspoon ground black pepper

Directions:

Preheat the oven to 350 degrees, Fahrenheit and precook the quinoa. Set it aside until ready to use.

Poke the squash with a fork or knife to let the steam out (and to avoid a squash explosion). Place on a microwave safe dish and microwave on high for three to four minutes. This will soften the squash before you cut into it.

Let the squash cool for five minutes and then cut it in half. Carefully remove the seeds as they will still be hot. Place the halves, cut side down, on a parchment-lined baking sheet. Bake for 30 to 40 minutes, until the squash is soft.

While squash is cooking, pour the water into a skillet over medium high heat and sauté the onion.

Reduce the heat to low and add the cloves, cardamom, ginger and cinnamon, stirring to mix. Turn off the heat and set the mixture aside until the squash is finished baking.

Once the squash is soft inside, remove it from the oven, but do not turn off the heat. As soon as it can be handled, carefully scoop the squash meat from the shell without damaging the skin. Mash the squash meat.

Add the squash meat to the onion spice mix in the skillet and turn the heat back on to medium high, stirring to mix.

Add the raisins and nuts and stir while heating through. Season with salt and pepper.

Turn off the heat and pack the shells with the mixture in the pan. Put the squash shells back on the baking sheet, cover everything with foil and bake for another 20 minutes before serving.

Spicy Corn and Spinach Casserole

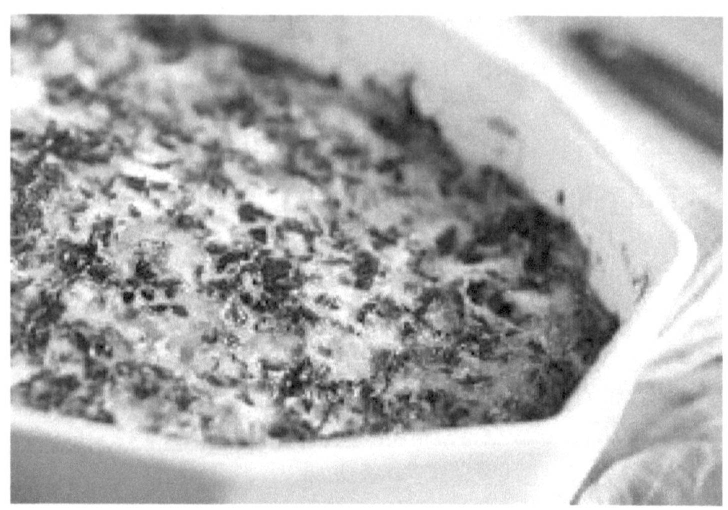

Preparation time: 10 minutes

Cooking time: 30 minutes

Servings: 4

Ingredients:

1½ cups water

¾ cup unsweetened soy milk, divided

1¼ cups cornmeal

1 14-ounce block tofu, drained and rinsed

3 cloves garlic, minced

1 10-ounce package frozen corn, thawed, divided

2 4.5-ounce cans mild chilies, diced

1 10-ounce package frozen spinach, thawed, with the liquid squeezed out

1 teaspoon baking powder

½ teaspoon cayenne pepper

½ teaspoon cumin

½ teaspoon salt

½ teaspoon pepper

Directions:

Preheat the oven to 450 degrees, Fahrenheit.

Heat the water and a half cup of the soy milk in a medium saucepan, bringing it almost to a boil. Turn off the burner and slowly whisk in the cornmeal, letting It thicken. Scrape out into a bowl and set it aside until ready to use.

Wrap the tofu in a paper towel and press down to extract most of the liquid. This may require repeating several times, with fresh paper towels.

When the tofu is as dry as you can get it, place it in a food processor, along with the garlic, one cup of corn and the remaining soy milk. Process until smooth, then pour it into the bowl with the cornmeal, folding it in to combine thoroughly.

To the same bowl, add the rest of the corn, the chilies, spinach, baking powder, cayenne pepper, cumin, salt and pepper. The mixture will be thick but needs to be combined well. Use your muscles.

Pour the mixture into an oiled baking dish and bake for 60 to 70 minutes. The edges should be crispy and the middle should jiggle just a little bit.

Let the casserole stand for 20 minutes before serving with salsa.

Steaks of Cauliflower With Pea Puree

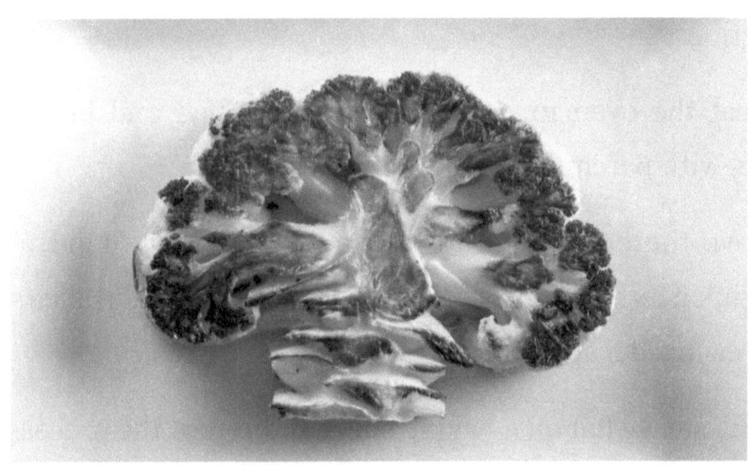

Preparation time: 10 minutes

Cooking time: 30 minutes

Servings: 4

Ingredients:

2 heads cauliflower

5 teaspoons olive oil, divided

½ teaspoon coriander

1 teaspoon paprika

¼ teaspoon black pepper

1 small onion, chopped

1 10-ounce bag frozen green peas

¼ cup unsweetened soy or almond milk

2 tablespoons fresh parsley, chopped

Directions:

Preheat the oven to 425 degrees, Fahrenheit and line baking sheets with parchment paper.

Remove the bottom core from the cauliflower. Stand a head upright on its base and cut it in half down the middle. Slice steaks from each side, about ¾-inch thick.

Lay the steaks flat on a baking sheet and repeat the process with the second head of cauliflower.

Brush two teaspoons of olive oil onto the steaks and sprinkle with the coriander, paprika and pepper. Flip the steaks do the same with the other side.

Bake for 15 minutes, then remove from the oven and flip the steaks over. Return them to the oven and bake for 15 more minutes.

While the steaks are baking, prepare the pea puree by placing a teaspoon of olive oil in a skillet over medium heat. Sauté the onion until it is translucent but do not let it brown.

Microwave the peas until they are plump and hot.

Place the onion, peas, soy milk and parsley in a blender and process until smooth.

Serve the puree, poured over the cauliflower steaks.

Thai Tofu With Peanut Butter Sauce

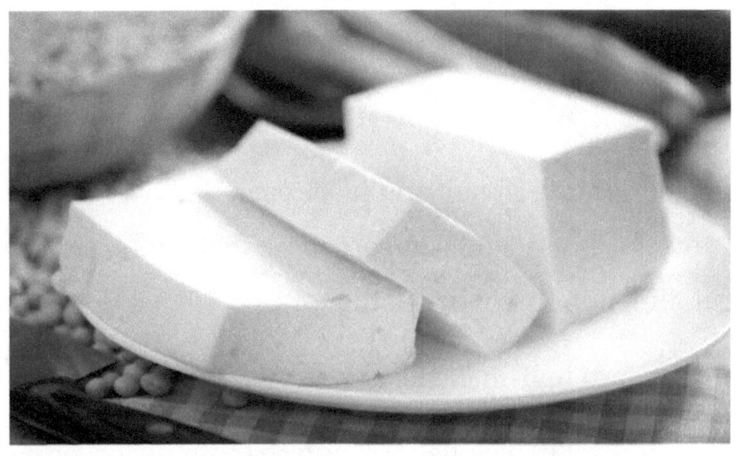

Preparation time: 10 minutes

Cooking time: 30 minutes

Servings: 4

Ingredients:

14-ounces firm tofu

1½ tablespoons olive oil

3½ teaspoons maple syrup

¼ cup rice vinegar

¼ cup warm water, ranging up to ½ cup

2 tablespoons fresh cilantro, finely chopped

3 cloves garlic, minced

1 teaspoon crushed red pepper flakes

1½ cups fresh spinach leaves, chopped

Prepared rice or quinoa for serving

Directions:

Cut the block of tofu in half and place each half between a couple paper towels. Press and squeeze both halves to remove any excess liquid, but do not break the tofu.

Cut the tofu into half-inch cubes

Place the olive oil in a skillet and add the tofu. Fry over medium heat, stirring gently until the tofu turns golden brown and the liquid in the pan has evaporated. Set the tofu aside, still in its pan.

In a bowl, whisk together the maple syrup, rice vinegar, soy sauce or tamari, a quarter cup of the warm water, the cilantro, garlic and red pepper flakes. Add the peanut butter and whisk until well combined. If it is too thick, add the rest of the warm water gradually, until it reaches the right consistency.

Place the skillet with the tofu back over low heat. Add the spinach and let it wilt.

Pour the peanut sauce over the mixture and simmer for five to 10 minutes. IF the sauce thickens too much, add more water to thin it.

Serve over rice or quinoa as desired.

Walnut Matzah Loaf

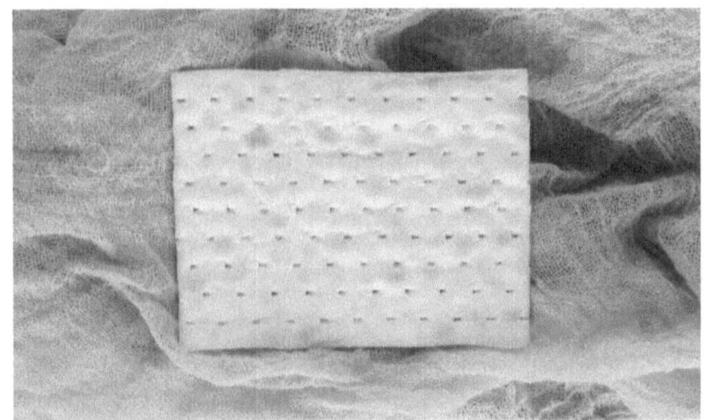

Preparation time: 10 minutes

Cooking time: 30 minutes

Servings: 4

Ingredients:

1 medium onion, finely chopped

1½ cups matzah meal or whole-grain breadcrumbs

1 cup ground walnuts

2 tablespoons fresh parsley, chopped

1 tablespoon egg replacer (powder)

1 tablespoon ground flaxseed

1 teaspoon salt

1½ cups unsweetened soy milk or other plant milk (I prefer almond milk)

Directions:

Line a standard loaf pan with parchment paper, extending it up the long sides of the pan in order to create handles you can use to lift the baked loaf out of the pan.

Heat the vegetable stock in a large skillet over medium heat. Add the onion and sauté until translucent.

In a bowl, combine the matzah or breadcrumbs, walnuts, parsley, egg replacer powder, flaxseed, salt and tomato paste; mix well.

Pour in the milk and sautéed onions and combine well. use your hands to mix everything together, then pack the mixture into the loaf pan.

Preheat the oven to 350 degrees, Fahrenheit and let the pan set for 30 minutes before placing it in the oven.

Bake for one hour, then remove the pan from the oven and let it set for 10 to 15 minutes.

Extract the loaf from the pan using the parchment handles, slice and serve.

Mexicrema

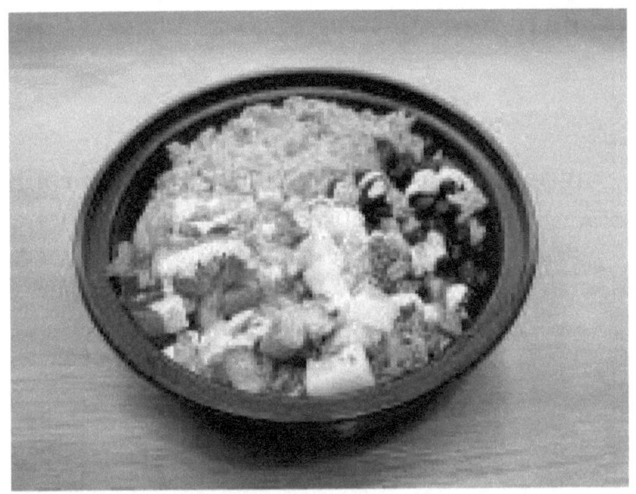

Preparation time: 10 minutes

Cooking time: 45 minutes

Servings: 4

Ingredients

1 cup silky firm organic tofu ("silken")

½ teaspoon garlic powder

½ teaspoon onion powder

Lemon or lime juice

2 tablespoons of water

¼ cup apple cider vinegar

2 tablespoons nutritional yeast

½ teaspoon of sea salt

1 handful fresh cilantro

¼ cup avocado (optional)

Directions

Mix all the ingredients in a blender until well incorporated.

Chile with "cheese" and sauce

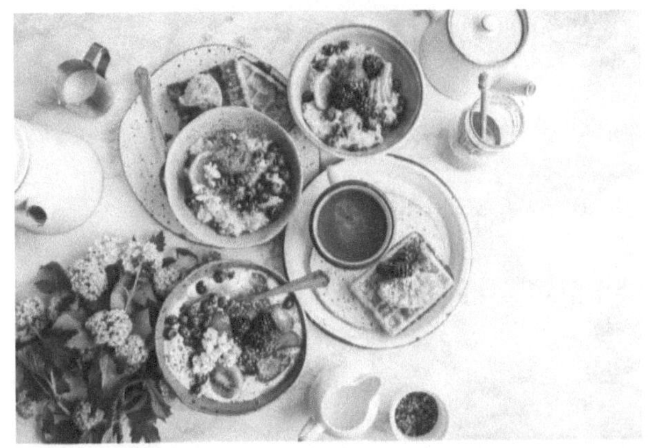

Preparation time: 10 minutes

Cooking time: 40 minutes

Servings: 4

1 cup raw cashews

2 red peppers, roasted, with the peel and seeds removed

¼ cup fresh lemon juice

3 tablespoons nutritional yeast

1 teaspoon salt

½ teaspoon red pepper in crushed flakes, or to taste

SAUCE

1 ½ cups diced tomato

½ cup diced bell pepper

¼ finely sliced red onion

½ teaspoon grated garlic

1 tablespoon fresh lemon juice

1 tablespoon chopped fresh cilantro

1 teaspoon jalapeño, seeded and chopped

Salt and fresh ground pepper

Directions

"CHEESE" UNTABLE

In a high-power blender, combine all the ingredients with two tablespoons of water and process everything until smooth.

SAUCE

In a medium bowl, combine all the ingredients on the list until jalapeño. Season everything with salt and pepper to taste.

Tomatillo green sauce

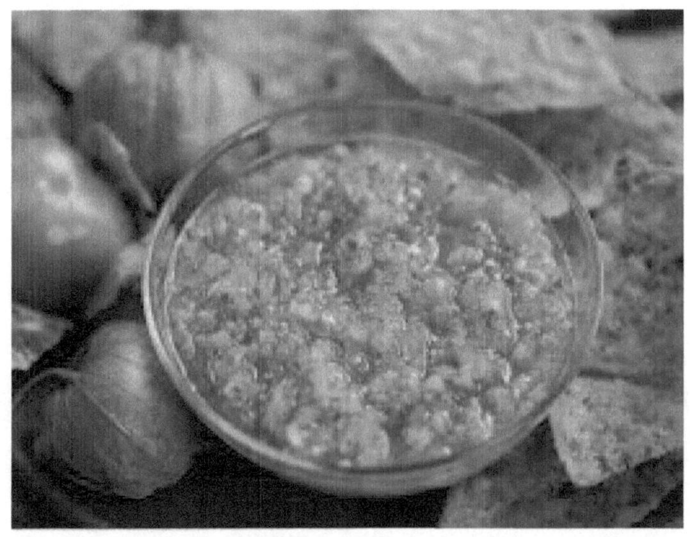

Preparation time: 10 minutes

Cooking time: 34 minutes

Servings: 4

Ingredients

8 small tomatillos (approximately 1 pound or 453 grams)

½ white onion, cut in half

1½ teaspoon ground garlic (approximately 3 small teeth)

1 jalapeño, cut in half and seeded

⅓ cup full of chopped cilantro

1 can (4 ounces or 113 grams) of chopped soft green chiles

OPTIONAL ADDITIONS

½ tablespoon ground cumin

Salt and pepper to taste

Jalapeño Seeds (to add spicily)

Directions

Preheat the grill. Cover a large baking sheet with foil.

Prepare the tomatillos: remove their lanterns, wash them, and cut them in half.

Place the tomatillos and onion upside down on the prepared baking sheet. Add the garlic and jalapeño to the tray.

Roast for five to seven minutes or until everything is uniformly charred.

In a blender or food processor, mix the charred ingredients, cilantro, and chiles until the sauce is smooth.

Matcha bars without baking with chocolate and coconut

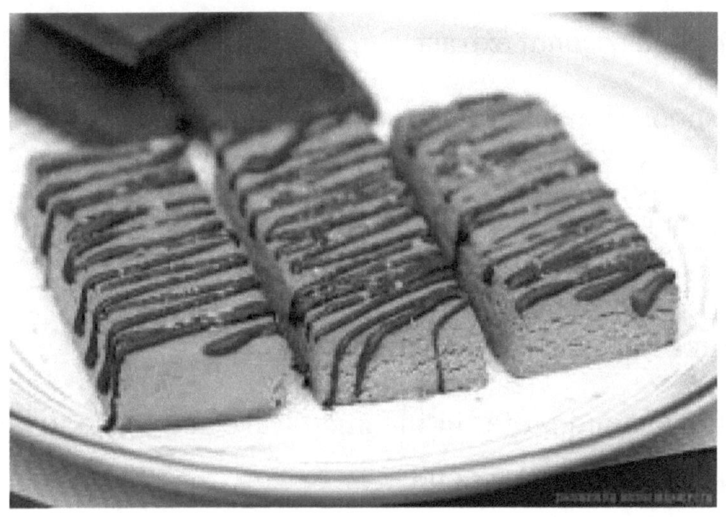

Preparation time: 10 minutes

Cooking time: 60 minutes

Servings: 4

Ingredients

1 cup oatmeal

½ cup raw cashews

⅓ cup coconut flour

½ cup nut butter

1 cup coconut milk lite

4 tablespoons matcha powder

2 tablespoons raw cocoa powder

2 tablespoons unsweetened coconut flakes

2 tablespoons maple syrup

½ teaspoon coconut extract

½ teaspoon cinnamon

Directions

Mix oats and cashews in a food processor

Place in a large bowl the mixture.

Melt the almond butter in the microwave and blend it with the mixture for about 30 seconds.

Add the remaining ingredients and mix well.

Cover a rectangular container or tray (preferably with some depth so that the bars are not too thin) with baking paper.

Add the mixture into the bowl. Flatten it as much as you can.

Sprinkle the dressings you want - I added a little more grated coconut and matcha to mine - but you can add some peanut butter, chocolate chips, nuts, etc.

cool the mixture for a few hours or until ready.

Cut it into bars and enjoy!

Chapter 12: Dinner

Lentil and Chickpea Salad

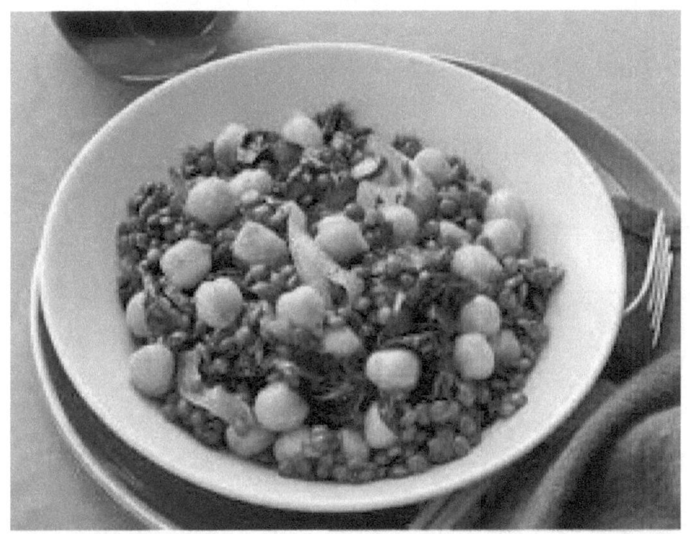

Preparation time: 10 minutes

Cooking time: 0 minute

Servings: 4

INGREDIENTS: For the Lemon Dressing:

¼ cup lemon juice

2 tablespoons olive oil

1 teaspoon Dijon mustard

1 teaspoon honey or maple syrup

½ teaspoon minced garlic

¼ teaspoon of sea salt

¼ teaspoon ground black pepper

For the Salad:

2 cups French green lentils, cooked

1 ½ cups cooked chickpeas

1 medium avocado, pitted, sliced

1 big bunch of radishes, chopped

¼ cup chopped mint and dill

Crumbled vegan feta cheese as needed

Direction

Prepare the dressing and for this, place all of its ingredients in a bowl and whisk until combined.

Take a large bowl, place all the ingredients for the salad in it, drizzle with the dressing and toss until combined.

Serve straight away.

Lebanese Bean Salad

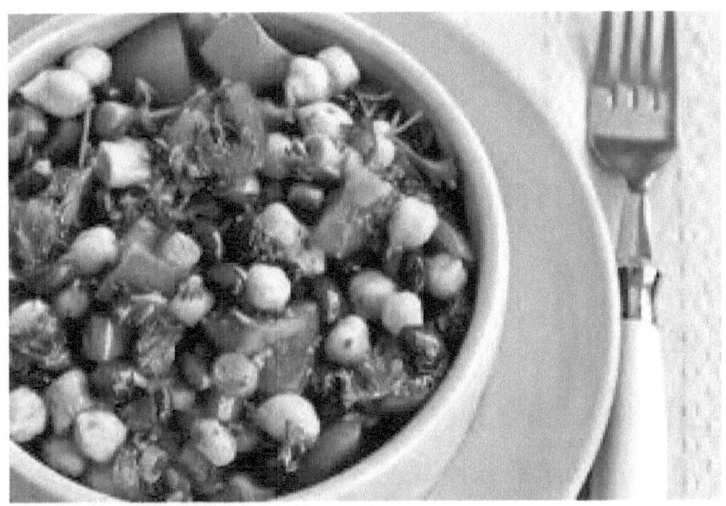

Preparation time: 10 minutes

Cooking time: 0 minute

Servings: 4

INGREDIENTS: For the Salad:

1 ½ cups cooked chickpeas

3 cups cooked kidney beans

1 small red onio n, peeled, diced

1 medium cucumber, peeled, deseeded, diced

2 stalks celery, chopped

¾ cup chopped parsley

2 tablespoons chopped dill

For the Dressing:

1 ½ teaspoon minced garlic

¾ teaspoon salt

¼ cup olive oil

1/8 teaspoon red pepper flakes

¼ cup lemon juice

Direction

Prepare the dressing and for this, place all of its ingredients in a bowl and whisk until combined.

Take a large bowl, place all the ingredients for the salad in it, drizzle with the dressing and toss until combined.

Serve straight away.

Roasted Carrots with Farro, and Chickpeas

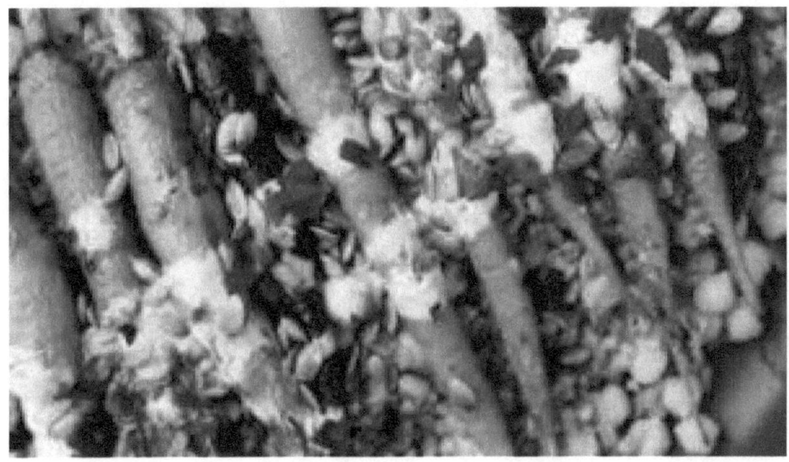

Preparation time: 10 minutes

Cooking time: 35 minutes

Servings: 4

INGREDIENTS: For the Chickpeas and Farro:

1 cup farro, cooked

1 ½ cups cooked chickpeas

½ teaspoon minced garlic

1 teaspoon lemon juice

½ teaspoon salt

1 teaspoon olive oil

For the Roasted Carrots:

1 pound heirloom carrots, scrubbed

½ teaspoon ground black pepper

¼ teaspoon ground cumin

1 teaspoon salt

1 tablespoon olive oil

For the Spiced Pepitas:

3 tablespoons green pumpkin seeds

1/8 teaspoon salt

1/8 teaspoon red chili powder

1/8 teaspoon cumin

½ teaspoon olive oil

For the Crème Fraiche:

1 tablespoon chopped parsley

1/3 cup vegan crème fraîche

¼ teaspoon ground black pepper

1/3 teaspoon salt

2 teaspoons water

For the Garnish:

1 more tablespoon chopped parsley

Direction

Prepare chickpeas and farro and for this, place all of its ingredients in a bowl and toss until combined.

Prepare the carrots and for this, arrange them on a baking sheet lined with parchment paper, drizzle with oil, sprinkle with the seasoning, toss until coated, and bake for 35 minutes until roasted and fork-tender, turning halfway.

Meanwhile, prepare pepitas and for this, take a skillet pan, place it over medium heat, add oil and when hot, add remaining ingredients in it and cook for 3 minutes until seeds are golden on the edges, set aside, and let it cool.

Prepare the crème Fraiche and for this, place all its ingredients in a bowl and whisk until combined.

Top chickpeas and farro with carrots, drizzle with crème Fraiche, sprinkle with pepitas and parsley and then serve.

Lentil Soup

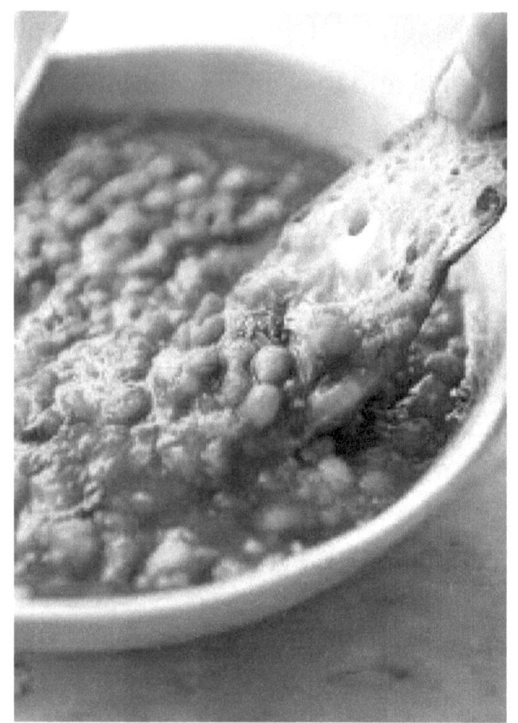

Preparation time: 10 minutes

Cooking time: 50 minutes

Servings: 4

Ingredients:

1 cup green lentils

1 medium white onion, peeled, chopped

1 cup chopped kale leaves

28 ounces diced tom atoes

2 carrots, peeled, chopped

2 teaspoons minced garlic

1 teaspoon curry powder

¼ teaspoon ground black pepper

1 teaspoon salt

2 teaspoons ground cumin

1/8 teaspoon red pepper flakes

½ teaspoon dried thyme

¼ cup olive oil

4 cups vegetable broth

1 tablespoon lemon juice

2 cups of water

Direction

Take a large pot, place it over medium heat, add 1 tablespoon oil and when hot, add onion and carrot and cook for 5 minutes until softened.

Then stir in garlic, curry powder, cumin and thyme, cook for 1 minute, then stir in tomatoes and cook for 3 minutes.

Add lentils, pour in water and broth, season with black pepper, salt, and red pepper and bring the mixture to a boil.

Switch heat to medium-low, simmer lentils for 30 minutes, then puree half of the soup, return it into the pan, stir in kale and cook for 5 minutes until softened.

Drizzle with lemon juice and serve straight away.

Spaghetti Squash Burrito Bowls

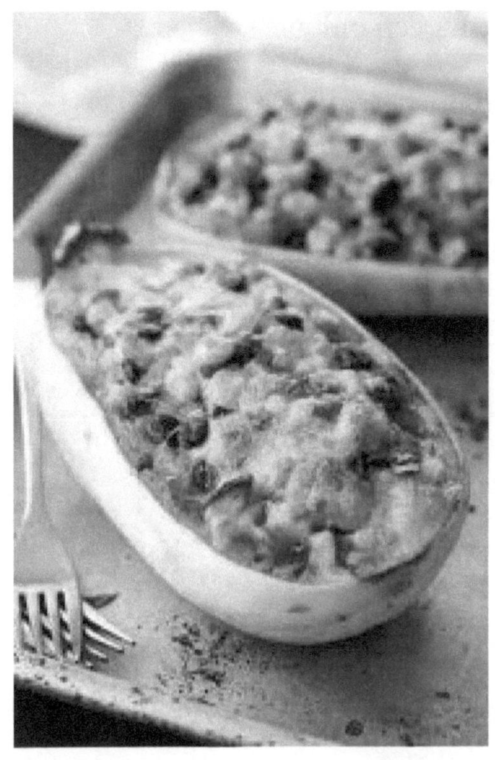

Preparation time: 10 minutes

Cooking time: 60 minutes

Servings: 4

INGREDIENTS: For the Spaghetti Squash:

2 medium spaghetti squas h , halved, deseeded

2 tablespoons olive oil

1 teaspoon salt

½ teaspoon ground black pepper

For the Slaw:

1/3 cup chopped green onions

2 cups chopped purple cabbage

1/3 cup chopped cilantro

15 ounces cooked black beans

1 medium red bell pepper, cored, chopped

¼ teaspoon salt

1 teaspoon olive oil

2 tablespoons lime juice

For the Salsa Verde:

1 avocado, pitted, diced

½ teaspoon minced garlic

¾ cup salsa verde

1/3 cup cilantro

1 tablespoon lime juice

Direction

Prepare the squash and for this, place squash halves on a baking sheet lined with parchment paper, rub them with oil, season with salt and black pepper and bake for 60 minutes until roasted and fork-tender.

Meanwhile, place the slaw and for this, place all of its ingredients in a bowl and toss until combined.

Prepare the salsa, and for this, place all of its ingredients in a food processor and pulse until smooth.

When squash has baked, fluff its flesh with a fork, then top with slaw and salsa and serve.

Quinoa and Black Beans

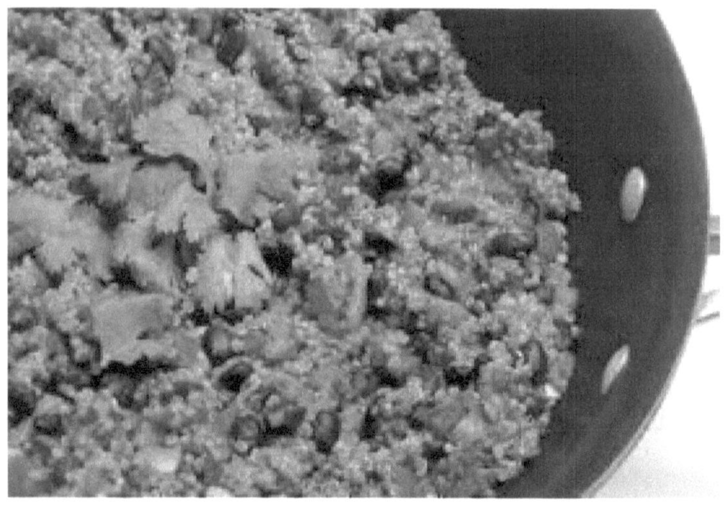

Preparation time: 10 minutes

Cooking time: 35 minutes

Servings: 4

Ingredients:

3/4 cup quinoa

30 ounces cooked black beans

1 medium white onion, peel ed, chopped

1 ½ teaspoon minced garlic

1 cup frozen corn kernels

¼ teaspoon ground black pepper

1/3 teaspoon salt

1 teaspoon ground cumin

1/4 teaspoon cayenne

1 teaspoon olive oil

1 1/2 cups vegetable broth

1/2 cup chopped cilantro

Direction

Take a saucepan, place it over medium heat, add oil and when hot, add onion and garlic, and cook for 10 minutes until softened.

Add quinoa, pour in the broth, stir in all the seasoning, then bring the mixture to a boil, switch heat to medium-low level and simmer for 20 minutes until the quinoa has absorbed all the liquid.

Add corn, stir until mixed, cook for 5 minutes until heated, and then stir in beans until mixed.

Garnish with cilantro and serve.

Spanish Rice

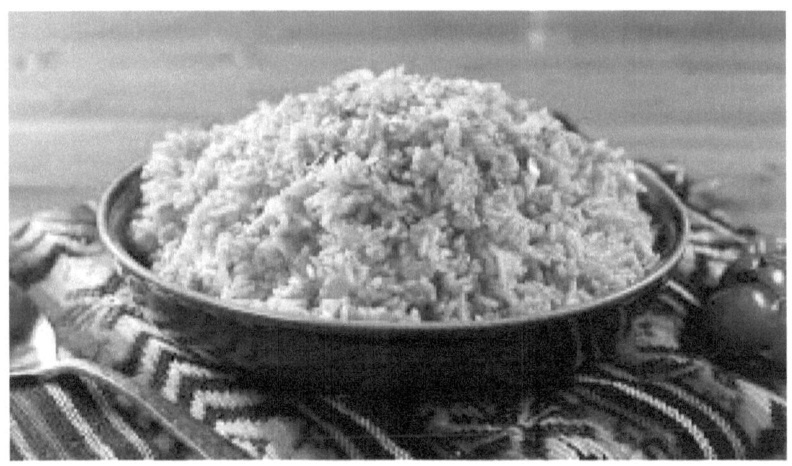

Preparation time: 5 minutes

Cooking time: 40 minutes

Servings: 4

Ingredients:

1/2 of medium green bell pepper, chopped

1 medium white onion, p eeled, chopped

10 ounces diced tomatoes with green chilies

1 teaspoon salt

2 teaspoons red chili powder

1 cup white rice

2 tablespoons olive oil

2 cups of water

Direction

Take a large skillet pan, place it over medium heat, add oil and when hot, add onion, pepper, and rice, and cook for 10 minutes.

Then add remaining ingredients, stir until mixed, bring the mixture to a boil, then simmer over medium-low heat for 30 minutes until cooked and most of the liquid has absorbed.

Serve straight away.

Stuffed Peppers

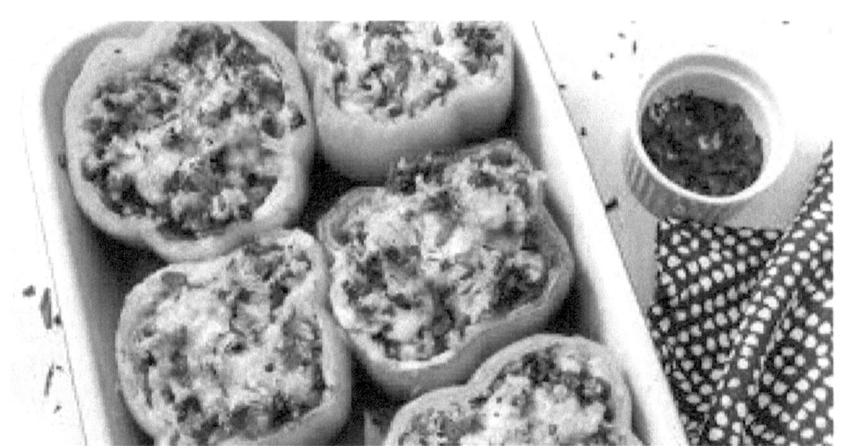

Preparation time: 10 minutes

Cooking time: 20 minutes

Servings: 4

Ingredients:

2 green onions, sliced

2 green bell peppers, halv ed, cored

1 large tomato, diced

1/2 cup Arborio rice, cooked

¼ teaspoon ground black pepper

1 teaspoon Italian seasoning

1 teaspoon salt

1 teaspoon dried basil

1 tablespoon olive oil

1 cup of water

1/2 cup crumbled vegan feta cheese

Direction

Prepare the peppers and for this, cut them in half, then remove the seeds and roast them on a greased baking sheet for 20 minutes at 400 degrees F until tender.

Meanwhile, heat oil in a skillet pan over medium-high heat and when hot, add onion, season with seasonings and herbs, and cook for 3 minutes.

Add tomatoes, stir well, cook for 5 minutes, then stir in rice and cook for 3 minutes until heated.

When done, remove the pan from heat, stir in cheese, and stuff the mixture into roasted peppers.

Serve straight away.

Black Beans and Rice

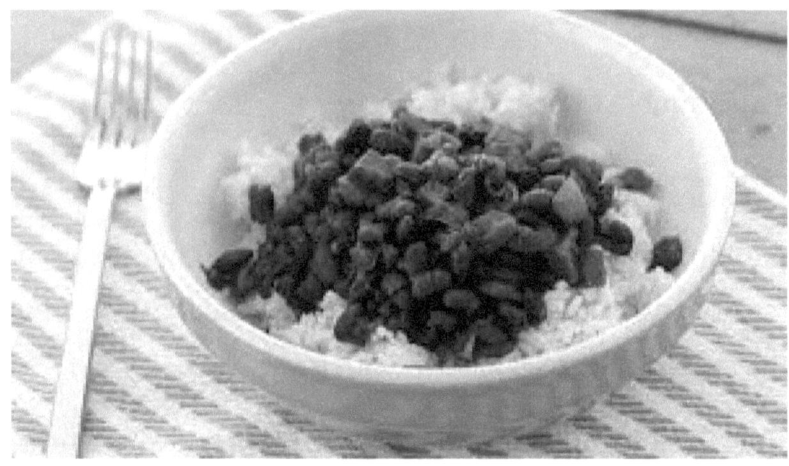

Preparation time: 10 minutes

Cooking time: 30 minutes

Servings: 4

Ingredients:

3/4 cup white rice

1 medium white onion, peeled, chopped

3 1/2 cups cooked black beans

1 teaspoon minced garlic

1/4 teaspoon cayenne pepper

1 teaspoon ground cumin

1 teaspoon olive oil

1 1/2 cups vegetable broth

Direction

Take a large pot over medium-high heat, add oil and when hot, add onion and garlic and cook for 4 minutes until saute.

Then stir in rice, cook for 2 minutes, pour in the broth, bring it to a boil, switch heat to the low level and cook for 20 minutes until tender.

Stir in remaining ingredients, cook for 2 minutes, and then serve straight away.

Vegetable Barley Soup

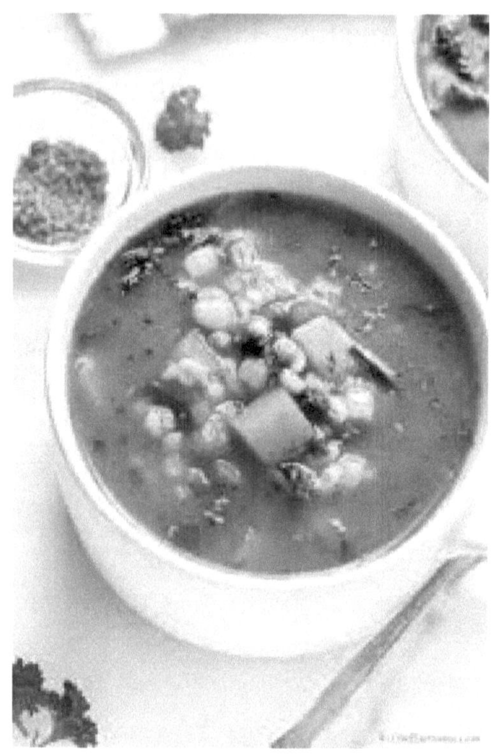

Preparation time: 5 minutes

Cooking time: 15 minutes

Servings: 8

Ingredients:

1 cup barley

14.5 ounces diced tomatoes wi th juice

2 large carrots, chopped

15 ounces cooked chickpeas

2 stalks celery, chopped

1 zucchini, chopped

1 medium white onion, peeled, chopped

1/2 teaspoon ground black pepper

1 teaspoon garlic powder

1 teaspoon curry powder

1 teaspoon salt

1 teaspoon paprika

1 teaspoon white sugar

1 teaspoon dried parsley

1 teaspoon Worcestershire sauce

3 bay leaves

2 quarts vegetable broth

Direction

Place all the ingredients in a pot, stir until mixed, place it over medium-high heat and bring the mixture to a boil.

Switch heat to medium level, simmer the soup for 90 minutes until cooked, and when done, remove bay leaf from it.

Serve straight away.

Lentils and Rice with Fried Onions

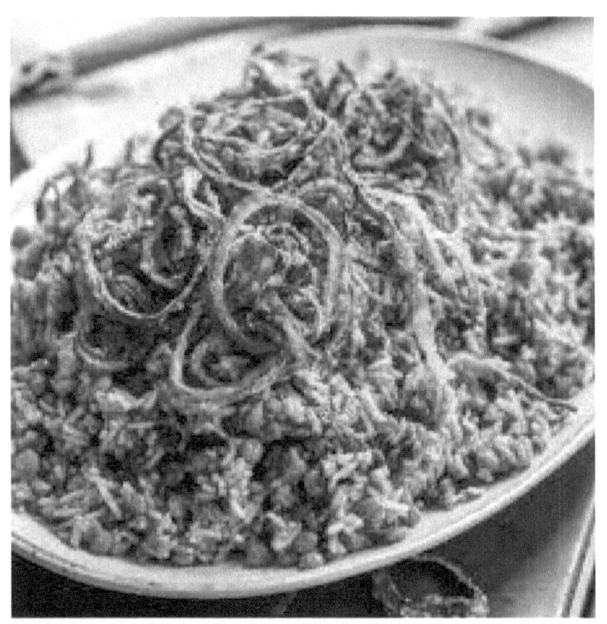

Preparation time: 5 minutes

Cooking time: 7 minutes

Servings: 4

Ingredients:

3/4 cup long-grain white rice, cooked

1 large white onion, peeled, sliced

1 1/3 cups green lentils, cooked

½ teaspoon salt

1/4 cup vegan sour cream

¼ teaspoon ground black pepper

6 tablespoons olive oil

Direction

Take a large skillet pan, place it over medium heat, add oil and when hot, add onions, and cook for 10 minutes until browned, set aside until required.

Take a saucepan, place it over medium heat, grease it with oil, add lentils and beans and cook for 3 minutes until warmed.

Season with salt and black pepper, cook for 2 minutes, then stir in half of the browned onions, and top with cream and remaining onions.

Serve straight away.

Asparagus Rice Pilaf

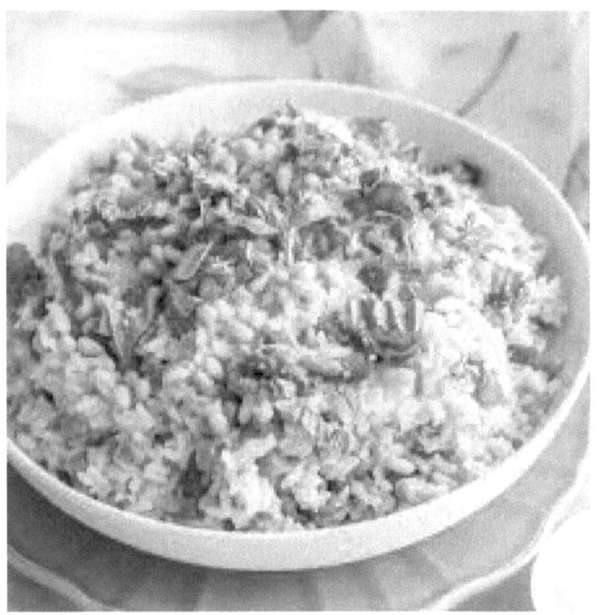

Preparation time: 10 minutes

Cooking time: 35 minutes

Servings: 4

Ingredients:

1 1/4 cups rice

1/2 pound asparagus, dice d, boiled

2 ounces spaghetti, whole-grain, broken

1/4 cup minced white onion

1/2 teaspoon minced garlic

1/2 cup cashew halves

¼ teaspoon ground black pepper

½ teaspoon salt

1/4 cup vegan butter

2 1/4 cups vegetable broth

Direction

Take a saucepan, place it over medium-low heat, add butter and when it melts, stir in spaghetti and cook for 3 minutes until golden brown.

Add onion and garlic, cook for 2 minutes until tender, then stir in rice, cook for 5 minutes, pour in the broth, season with salt and black pepper and bring it to a boil.

Switch heat to medium level, cook for 20 minutes, then add cashews and asparagus and stir until combined.

Serve straight away.

Mexican Stuffed Peppers

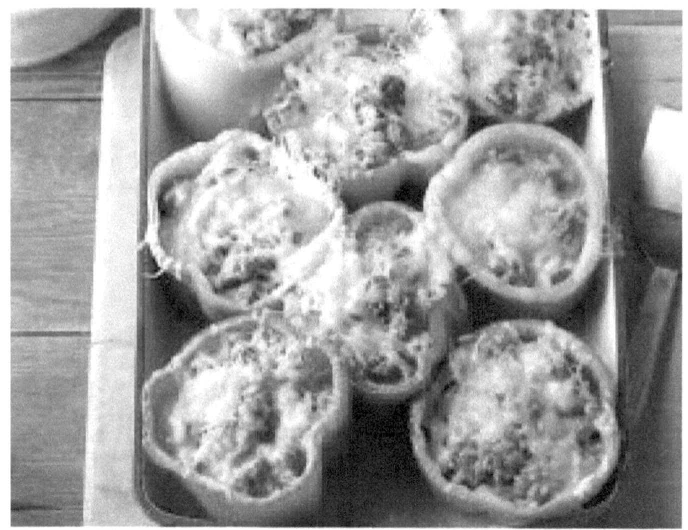

Preparation time: 10 minutes

Cooking time: 40 minutes

Servings: 4

Ingredients:

2 cups cooked rice

1/2 cup chopped onion

15 ounces cooked black bean s

4 large green bell peppers, destemmed, cored

1 tablespoon olive oil

1 tablespoon salt

14.5 ounce diced tomatoes

1/2 teaspoon ground cumin

1 teaspoon garlic salt

1 teaspoon red chili powder

1/2 teaspoon salt

2 cups shredded vegan Mexican cheese blend

Direction

Boil the bell peppers in salty water for 5 minutes until softened and then set aside until required.

Heat oil over medium heat in a skillet pan, then add onion and cook for 10 minutes until softened.

Transfer the onion mixture in a bowl, add remaining ingredients, reserving ½ cup cheese blended, stir until mixed, and then fill this mixture into the boiled peppers.

Arrange the peppers in the square baking dish, sprinkle them with remaining cheese and bake for 30 minutes at 350 degrees F.

Serve straight away.

Mushroom Risotto

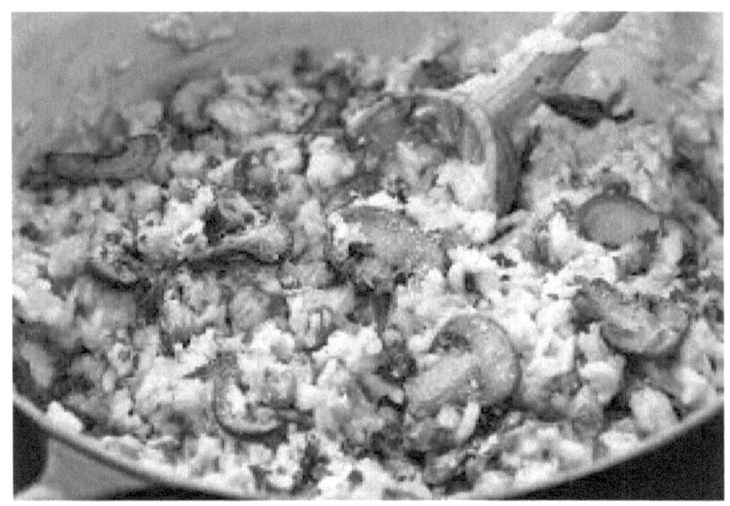

Preparation time: 10 minutes

Cooking time: 35 minutes

Servings: 4

Ingredients:

1 cup of rice

3 small white onions, peeled, chopped

1 teaspoon minced celery

1 ½ cups sliced mushrooms

½ teaspoon minced garlic

1 teaspoon minced parsley

½ teaspoon salt

¼ teaspoon ground black pepper

1 tablespoon olive oil

1 teaspoon vegan butter

¼ cup vegan cashew cream

1 cup grated vegan Parmesan cheese

1 cup of coconut milk

5 cups vegetable stock

Direction

Take a large skillet pan, place it over medium-high heat, add oil and when hot, add onion and garlic, and cook for 5 minutes.

Transfer to a plate, add celery and parsley into the pan, stir in salt and black pepper, and cook for 3 minutes.

Then switch heat to medium-low level, stir in mushrooms, cook for 5 minutes, then pour in cream and milk, stir in rice until combined, and bring the mixture to simmer.

Pour in vegetable stock, one cup at a time until it has absorbed and, when done, stir in cheese and butter.

Serve straight away.

Quinoa with Chickpeas and Tomatoes

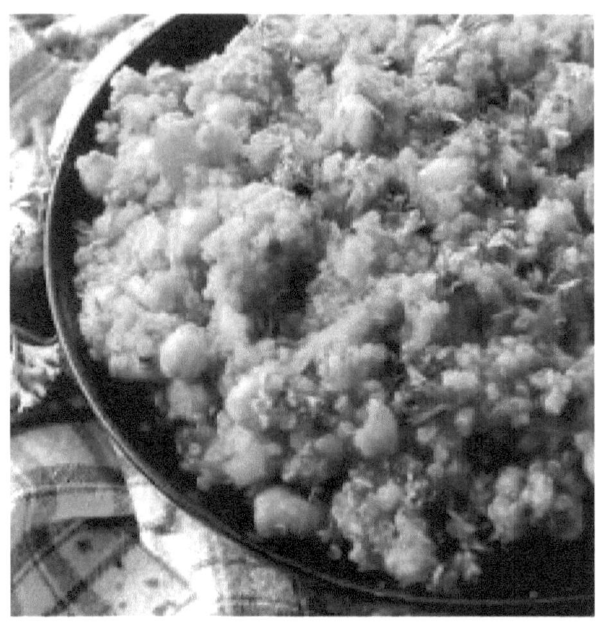

Preparation time: 10 minutes

Cooking time: 0 minute

Servings: 6

Ingredients:

1 tomato, chopped

1 cup quinoa, cooked

½ teaspoon minced garlic

¼ teaspoon ground black pepper

½ teaspoon salt

1/2 teaspoon ground cumin

4 teaspoons olive oil

3 tablespoons lime juice

1/2 teaspoon chopped parsley

Direction

Take a large bowl, place all the ingredients in it, except for the parsley, and stir until mixed.

Garnish with parsley and serve straight away.

Barley Bake

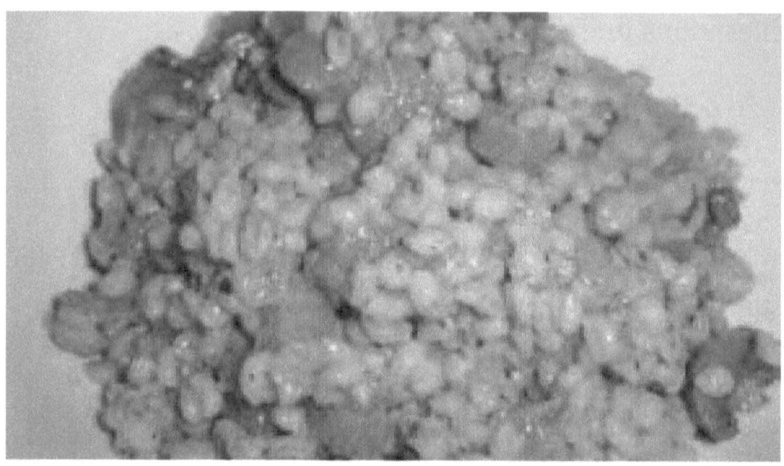

Preparation time: 10 minutes

Cooking time: 98 minutes

Servings: 6

Ingredients:

1 cup pearl barley

1 medium white onion, peeled, diced

2 green onions, sliced

1/2 cup sliced mushrooms

1/8 teaspoon ground black pepper

1/4 teaspoon salt

1/2 cup chopped parsley

1/2 cup pine nuts

1/4 cup vegan butter

29 ounces vegetable broth

Direction

Place a skillet pan over medium-high heat, add butter and when it melts, stir in onion and barley, add nuts and cook for 5 minutes until light brown.

Add mushrooms, green onions and parsley, sprinkle with salt and black pepper, cook for 1 minute and then transfer the mixture into a casserole dish.

Pour in broth, stir until mixed and bake for 90 minutes until barley is tender and has absorbed all the liquid.

Serve straight away.

Zucchini Risotto

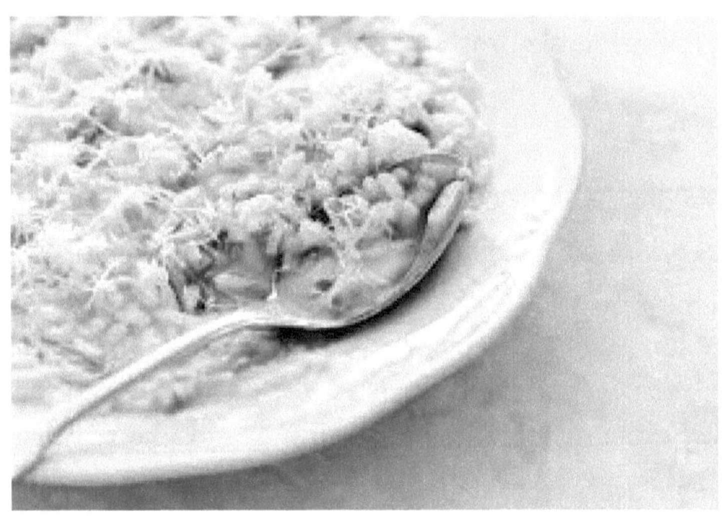

Preparation time: 10 minutes

Cooking time: 30 minutes

Servings: 6

Ingredients:

2 cups Arborio rice

10 sun-dried tomatoes, chopped

1 medium white onion, peeled, chopped

1 tablespoon chopped basil leaves

1/2 medium zucchini, sliced

1 teaspoon dried thyme

1/3 teaspoon ground black pepper

1 tablespoon vegan butter

6 tablespoons grated vegan Parmesan cheese

7 cups vegetable broth, hot

Direction

Take a large pot, place it over medium heat, add butter and when it melts, add onion and cook for 2 minutes.

Stir in rice, cook for another 2 minutes until toasted, and then stir in broth, 1 cup at a time until absorbed completely and creamy mixture comes together.

Then stir in remaining ingredients until combined, taste to adjust seasoning and serve.

Mushroom, Lentil, and Barley Stew

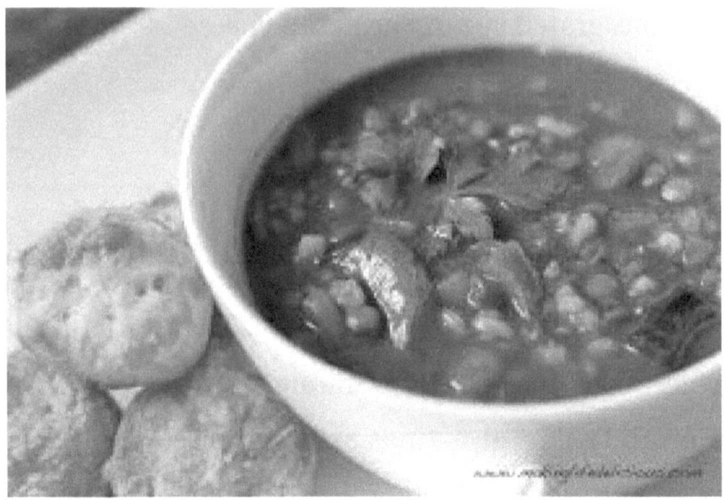

Preparation time: 10 minutes

Cooking time: 6 hours

Servings: 8

Ingredients:

3/4 cup pearl barley

2 cups sliced button mushrooms

3/4 cup dry lentils

1 ounce dried shiitake mushrooms

2 teaspoons minced garlic

1/4 cup dried onion flakes

2 teaspoons ground black pepper

1 teaspoon dried basil

2 ½ teaspoons salt

2 teaspoons dried savory

3 bay leaves

2 quarts vegetable broth

Direction

Switch on the slow cooker, place all the ingredients in it, and stir until combined.

Shut with lid and cook the stew for 6 hours at a high heat setting until cooked.

Serve straight away.

Tomato Barley Soup

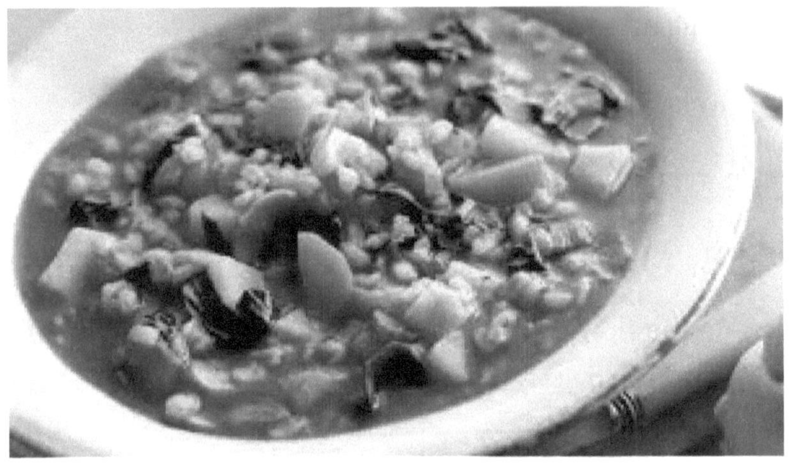

Preparation time: 10 minutes

Cooking time: 40 minutes

Servings: 6

Ingredients:

1/4 cup barley

1 cup chopped celery

14.5 ounces peeled and diced tomatoes

1 cup chopped white onions

2 tomatoes, diced

1 cup chopped carrots

2 teaspoons minced garlic

1/8 teaspoon ground black pepper

1 teaspoon salt

2 tablespoons olive oil

2 1/2 cups water

10.75 ounces chicken broth

Direction

Take a large saucepan, place it over medium heat, add onion, carrot, and celery, stir in garlic and cook for 10 minutes until tender.

Then add remaining ingredients, stir until combined, and bring the mixture to a boil.

Switch heat to the level, simmer the soup for 40 minutes and then serve straight away.

Black Beans, Corn, and Yellow Rice

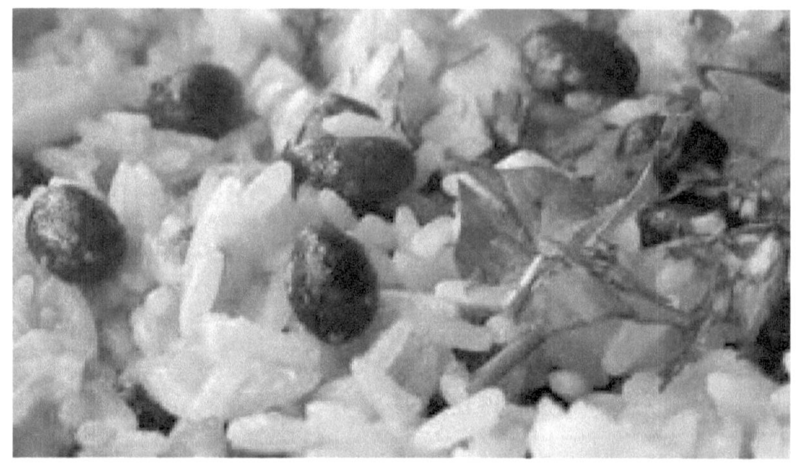

Preparation time: 10 minutes

Cooking time: 25 minutes

Servings: 8

Ingredients:

8 ounces yellow rice mix

15.25 ounces cooked kernel corn

1 1/4 cups water

15 ounces cooked black beans

1 teaspoon ground cumin

2 teaspoons lime juice

2 tablespoons olive oil

Direction

Place a saucepan over high heat, add oil, water, and rice, bring the mixture to a bowl, and then switch heat to medium-low level.

Simmer for 25 minutes until rice is tender and all the liquid has been absorbed and then transfer the rice to a large bowl.

Add remaining ingredients into the rice, stir until mixed and serve straight away.

Lemony Quinoa

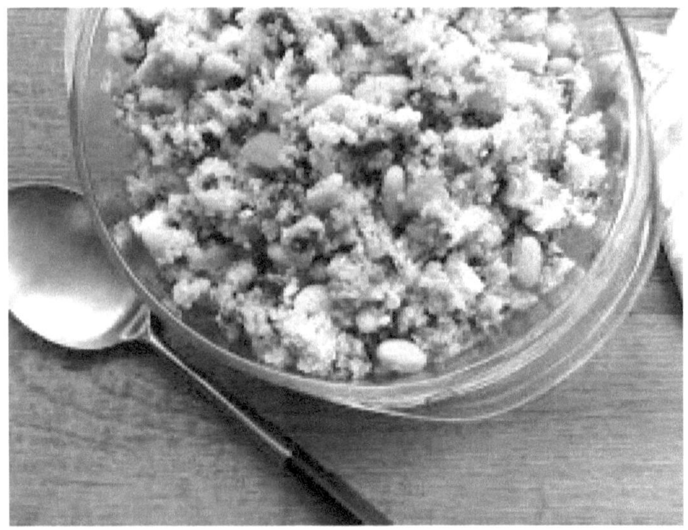

Preparation time: 10 minutes

Cooking time: 0 minute

Servings: 6

Ingredients:

1 cup quinoa, cooked

1/4 of medium red onion, p eeled, chopped

1 bunch of parsley, chopped

2 stalks of celery, chopped

¼ teaspoon of sea salt

1/4 teaspoon cayenne pepper

1/2 teaspoon ground cumin

1/4 cup lemon juice

1/4 cup pine nuts, toasted

Direction

Take a large bowl, place all the ingredients in it, and stir until combined.

Serve straight away.

Cuban Beans and Rice

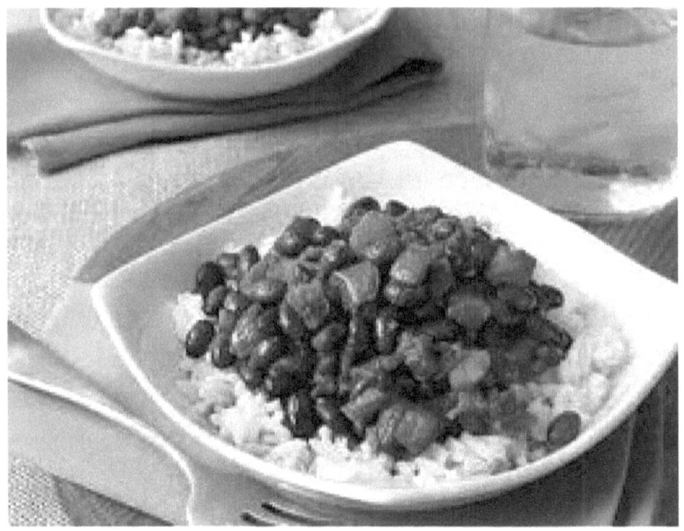

Preparation time: 10 minutes

Cooking time: 55 minutes

Servings: 6

Ingredients:

1 cup uncooked white rice

1 green bell pepper, cored, chopped

15.25 ounces cooked kidney beans

1 cup chopped white onion

4 tablespoons tomato paste

1 teaspoon minced garlic

1 teaspoon salt

1 tablespoon olive oil

2 ½ cups vegetable broth

Direction

Take a saucepan, place it over medium heat, add oil and when hot, add onion, garlic and bell pepper and cook for 5 minutes until tender.

Then stir in salt and tomatoes, switch heat to the low level and cook for 2 minutes.

Then stir in rice and beans, pour in the broth, stir until mixed and cook for 45 minutes until rice has absorbed all the liquid.

Serve straight away.

Beans Curry

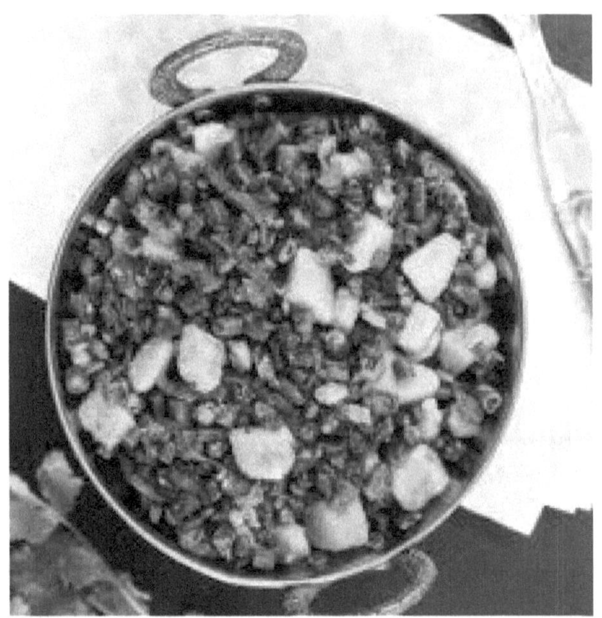

Preparation time: 10 minutes

Cooking time: 8 hours and 10 minutes

Servings: 5

Ingredients:

2 cups kidney beans, dried, soaked

1-inch of ginger, grated

1 ½ cup diced tomatoes

1 medium red onion, pe eled, sliced

1 tablespoon tomato paste

1 teaspoon minced garlic

1 small bunch cilantro, chopped

½ teaspoon cumin powder

1 teaspoon salt

1 ½ teaspoon curry powder

2 tablespoons olive oil

2 tablespoons lemon juice

Direction

Place onion in a food processor, add ginger and garlic, and pulse for 1 minute until blended.

Take a skillet pan, place it over medium heat, add oil and when hot, add the onion-garlic mixture, and cook for 5 minutes until softened and light brown.

Then add tomatoes and tomato paste, stir in ½ teaspoon salt, cumin and curry powder and cook for 5 minutes until cooked.

Drain the soaked beans, add them to the slow cooker, add cooked tomato mixture, and remaining ingredients except for cilantro and lemon juice and stir until mixed.

Switch on the slow cooker, then shut with lid and cook for 8 hours at high heat setting until tender.

When done, transfer 1 cup of beans to the blender, process until creamy, then return it into the slow cooker and stir until mixed.

Drizzle with lemon juice, top with cilantro, and serve.

Pasta with Kidney Bean Sauce

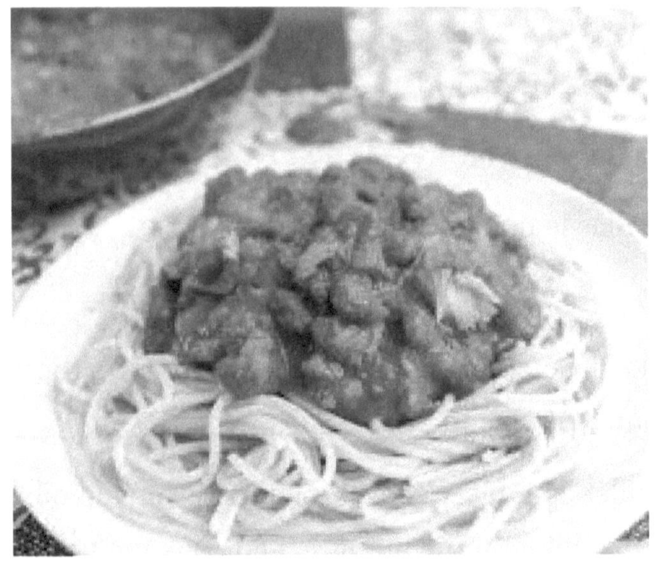

Preparation time: 5 minutes

Cooking time: 15 minutes

Servings: 4

Ingredients:

12 ounces cooked kidney beans

7 ounces whole-wheat pa sta, cooked

1 medium white onion, peeled, diced

1 cup arugula

2 tablespoons tomato paste

1 teaspoon minced garlic

½ teaspoon smoked paprika

1 teaspoon dried oregano

½ teaspoon cayenne pepper

1/3 teaspoon ground black pepper

2/3 teaspoon salt

2 tablespoons balsamic vinegar

Direction

Take a large skillet pan, place it over medium-high heat, add onion and garlic, splash with some water and cook for 5 minutes.

Then add remaining ingredients, except for pasta and arugula, stir until mixed and cook for 10 minutes until thickened.

When done, mash with the fork, top with arugula and serve with pasta.

Serve straight away

Stuffed Peppers with Kidney Beans

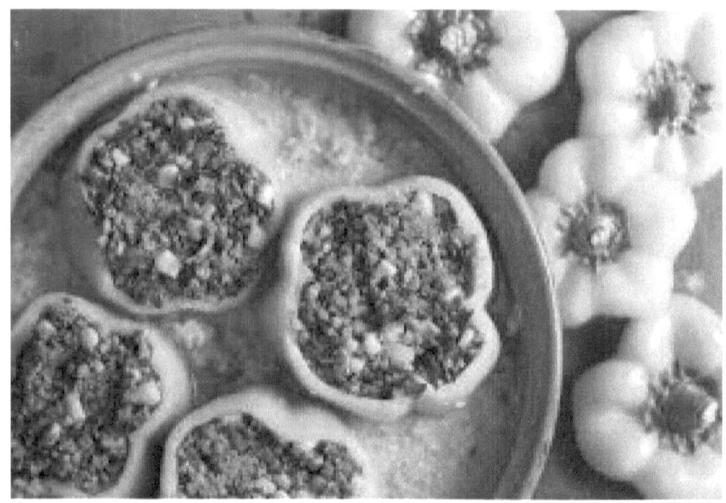

Preparation time: 5 minutes

Cooking time: 35 minutes

Servings: 4

Ingredients:

3.5 ounces cooked kidney beans

1 big tomato, diced

3.5 ounces sweet corn, canned

2 medium bell peppers, deseeded, halved

½ of medium red onion, peeled, diced

1 teaspoon garlic powder

1/3 teaspoon ground black pepper

2/3 teaspoon salt

½ teaspoon dried basil

3 teaspoons parsley

½ teaspoon dried thyme

3 tablespoons cashew

1 teaspoon olive oil

Direction

Switch on the oven, then set it to 400 degrees F and let it preheat.

Take a large skillet pan, place it over medium heat, add oil and when hot, add onion and cook for 2 minutes until translucent.

Add beans, tomatoes, and corn, stir in garlic and cashews and cook for 5 minutes.

Stir in salt, black pepper, parsley, basil, and thyme, remove the pan from heat and evenly divide the mixture between bell peppers.

Bake the peppers for 25 minutes until tender, then top with parsley and serve.

Nutrition Value:

Chickpea Shakshuka

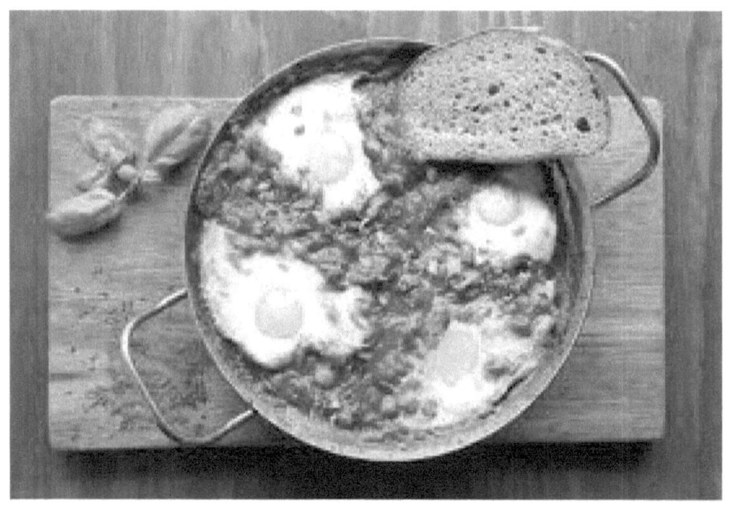

Preparation time: 5 minutes

Cooking time: 30 minutes

Servings: 6

Ingredients:

22 ounces cooked chickpeas

1/2 cup diced white onion

5 green olives

1/2 medium red bell pepper, chopped

1 1/2 Tbsp minced garlic

1 Tbsp coconut sugar

2 teaspoons red chili powder

2 teaspoons smoked paprika

1/8 teaspoon cayenne pepper

1 teaspoon salt

3 Tbsp tomato paste

1 tsp ground cumin

1/4 teaspoon ground cinnamon

1/8 teaspoon cardamom

1/8 teaspoon coriander

28-ounces tomato puree

1 Tbsp avocado oil

Direction

Take a large skillet pan, place it over medium heat, add oil and when hot, add garlic, onion and bell pepper and cook for 5 minutes until fragrant.

Then stir in the tomato puree and tomato paste, stir in all the spices until combined, bring the mixture to simmer, and cook for 3 minutes.

Add olives and chickpeas, stir to combine, switch heat to medium-low level and simmer for 20 minutes until cooked.

Serve straight away.

Thai Tofu

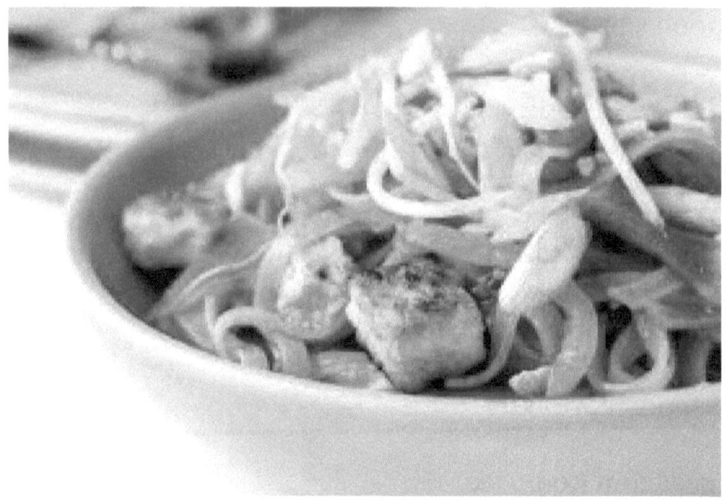

Preparation time: 5 minutes

Cooking time: 7 minutes

Servings: 4

Ingredients:

14 ounces tofu, firm, drained, 3/4 inch cubed

1/3 cup chopped green onion

2 teaspoons grated ginge r

3 tablespoons coconut flakes

1 teaspoon soy sauce

1 ½ teaspoon olive oil

¼ cup peanut butter

½ teaspoon sesame oil

1 teaspoon sesame seeds

Direction

Take a skillet pan, place it over medium-high heat. Reduce heat to medium, add both oils and when hot, add green onions and cook for 1 minute.

Then add tofu cubes, cook for 4 minutes and stir in soy sauce halfway.

Stir in ginger and peanut butter, stir gently until well incorporated, and then remove the pan from heat.

Sprinkle with sesame seeds and serve.

Chapter 13: Dessert and Snacks

Garlicky Kale Chips

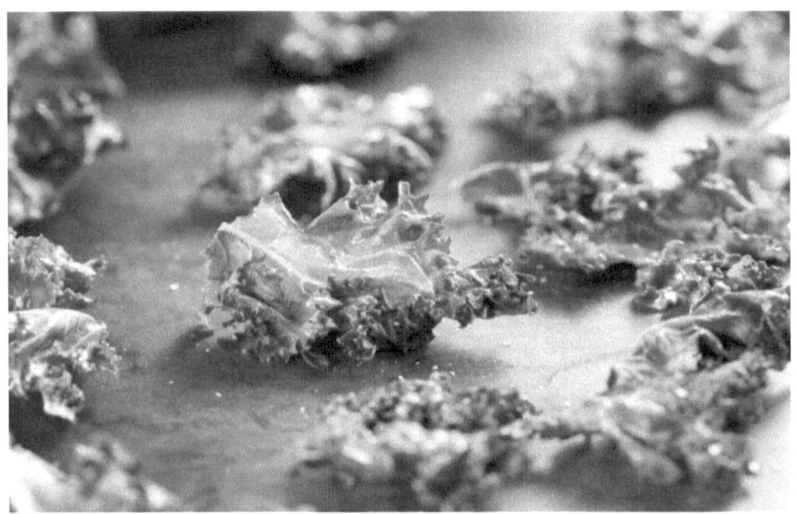

Preparation time: 5 minutes

Cooking time: 7 minutes

Servings: 4

Ingredients:

4 cloves garlic

1 cup olive oil

8 to 10 cups fresh kale, chopped

1 tablespoon of garlic-flavored olive oil

½ teaspoon garlic salt

½ teaspoon pepper

1 pinch red pepper flakes (optional)

Directions:

Peel and crush the garlic clove and place it in a small jar with a lid. Pour the olive oil over the top, cover tightly and shake. This will keep in the refrigerator for several days. When you're ready to use it, strain out the garlic and retain the oil.

Preheat the oven to 175 degrees, Fahrenheit.

Spread out the kale on a baking sheet and drizzle with the olive oil. Sprinkle with garlic salt, pepper and red pepper flakes.

Bake for an hour, remove from the oven and let the chips cool.

Store in an airtight container if you don't plan to eat them right away.

Hummus-stuffed Baby Potatoes

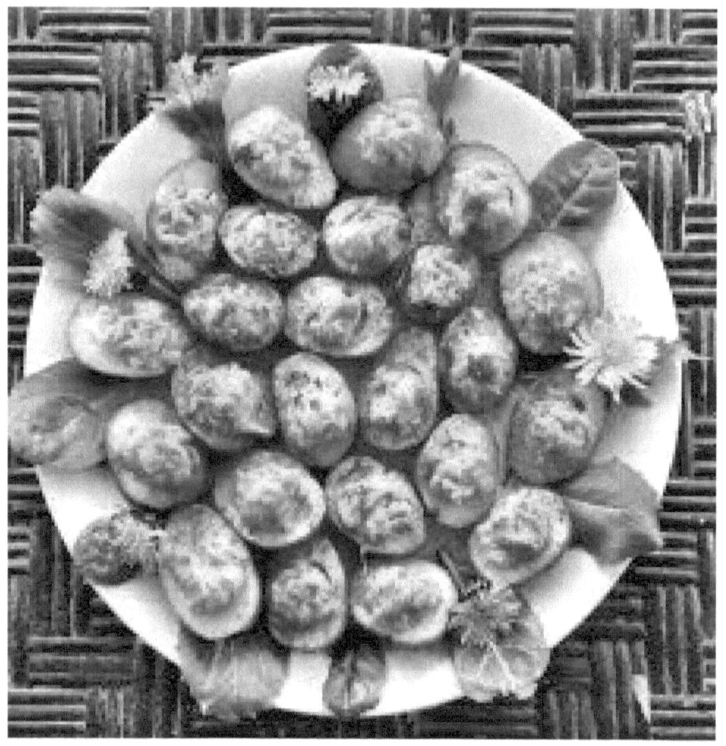

Preparation time: 10 minutes

Cooking time: 30 minutes

Servings: 4

Ingredients:

12 small red potatoes, walnut-sized or slightly larger

2 green onions, thinly sliced

¼ teaspoon paprika, for garnish

Directions:

Place two to three inches of water in a saucepan, set a steamer inside and bring the water to a boil.

Place the whole potatoes in the steamer basket and steam for about 20 minutes or until soft. Keep the pan from boiling dry by adding additional hot water as needed.

Dump the potatoes into a colander and run cold water over them until they can be handled.

Cut each potato open and scoop out most of the pulp, leaving the skin and a thin layer of potato intact.

Mix the hummus with most of the green onions (keep enough for garnish) and spoon a little into the area where the potato has been scooped out.

Sprinkle each filled potato half with paprika and serve.

Homemade Trail Mix

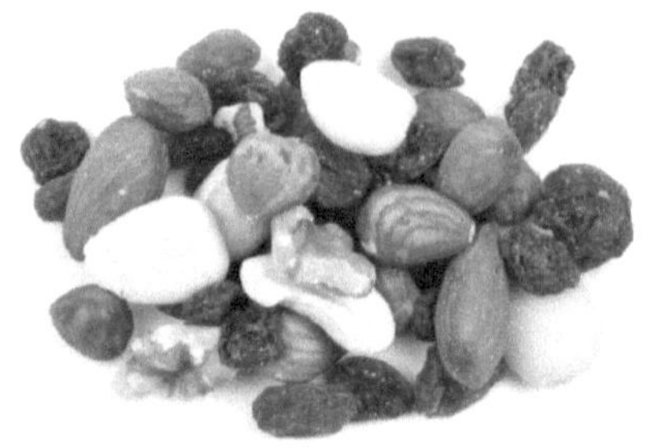

Preparation time: 5 minutes

Cooking time: 8 minutes

Servings: 4

Ingredients:

½ cup uncooked old-fashioned oatmeal

½ cup chopped dates

2 cups whole grain cereal

¼ cup raisins

¼ cup almonds

¼ cup walnuts

Directions:

Mix all the ingredients in a large bowl.

Place in an airtight container until ready to use.

Nut Butter Maple Dip

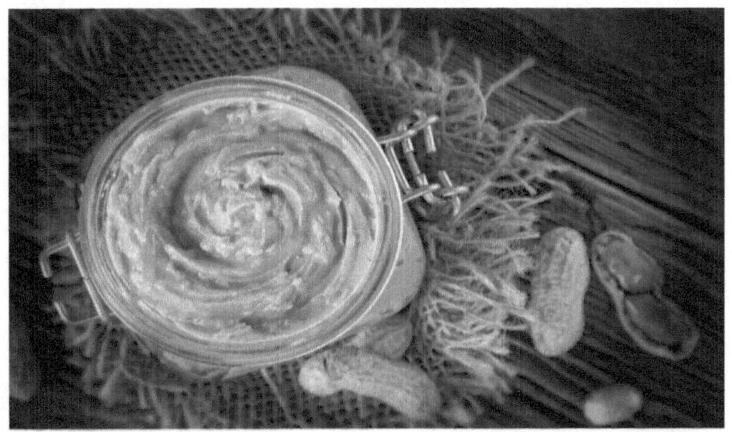

Preparation time: 5 minutes

Cooking time: 20 minutes

Servings: 4

Ingredients:

½ tablespoon ground flaxseed

1 teaspoon ground cinnamon

½ tablespoon maple syrup

2 tablespoons cashew milk

Directions:

In a bowl, combine the flaxseed, cinnamon, maple syrup, cashew milk and peanut butter.

Use a fork to mix everything in. I stir it like I'm scrambling eggs. The mixture should be creamy. If it's too runny, add a little more peanut butter; if it's too thick, add a little more cashew milk.

Refrigerate for about an hour, covered and serve.

Oven Baked Sesame Fries

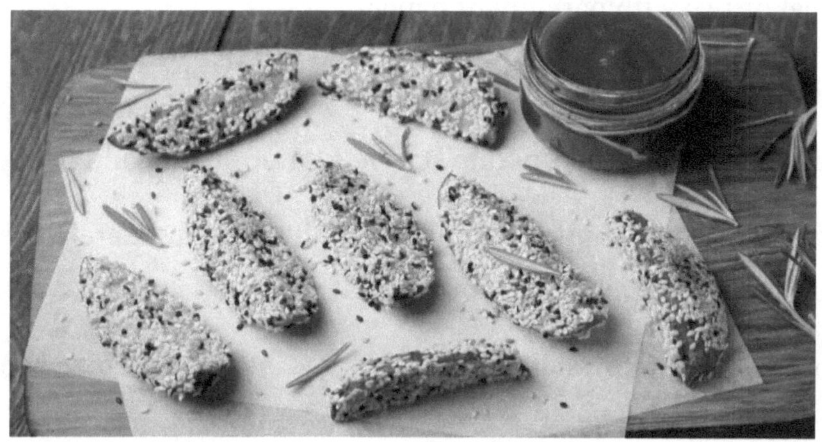

Preparation time: 5 minutes

Cooking time: 7 minutes

Servings: 4

Ingredients:

1 pound Yukon Gold potatoes, skins on and cut into wedges

2 tablespoons sesame seeds

1 tablespoon potato starch

1 tablespoon sesame oil

Salt to taste

Black pepper to taste

Directions:

Preheat the oven to 425 degrees, Fahrenheit and cover a baking sheet or two with parchment paper.

Cut the potatoes and place in a large bowl.

Add the sesame seeds, potato starch, sesame oil, salt and pepper.

Toss with your hands and make sure all the wedges are coated. Add more sesame seeds or oil if needed.

Spread the potato wedges on the baking sheets with some room between each wedge.

Bake for 15 minutes, flip the wedges over and then return them to the oven for 10 to 15 more minutes, until they look golden and crispy.

Pumpkin Orange Spice Hummus

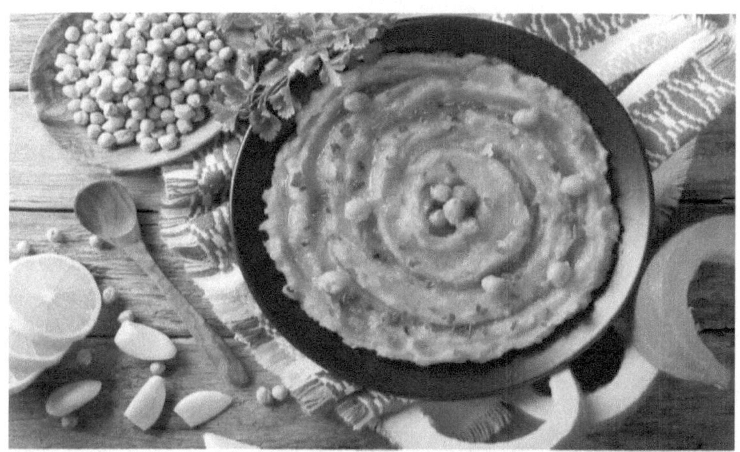

Preparation time: 5 minutes

Cooking time: 10 minutes

Servings: 4

Ingredients:

1 16-ounce can garbanzo beans, rinsed and drained

1 tablespoon apple cider vinegar

1 tablespoon maple syrup

¼ cup tahini

1 tablespoon fresh orange juice

½ teaspoon orange zest and additional zest for garnish

⅛ teaspoon ground cinnamon

⅛ teaspoon ground ginger

⅛ teaspoon ground nutmeg

¼ teaspoon salt

Directions:

Pour the pumpkin puree and garbanzo beans into a food processor and pulse to break up.

Add the vinegar, syrup, tahini, orange juice and orange zest pulse a few times.

Add the cinnamon, ginger, nutmeg and salt and process until smooth and creamy.

Serve in a bowl sprinkled with more orange zest with wheat crackers alongside.

Quick English Muffin Mexican Pizzas

Half An English Muffin Makes A Good Pizza Base

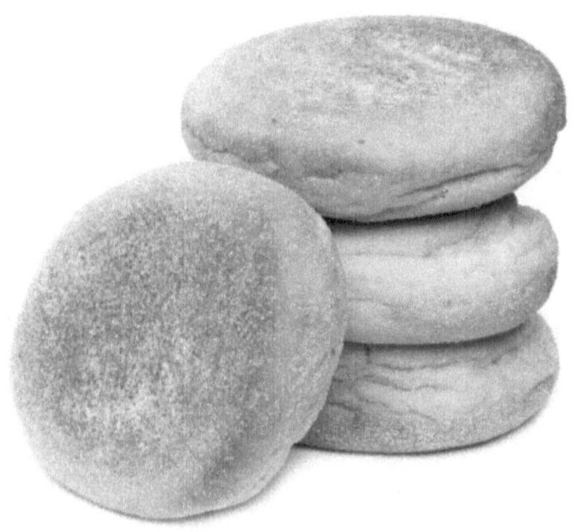

Preparation time: 5 minutes

Cooking time: 7 minutes

Servings: 4

Ingredients:

2 whole-wheat English muffins separated

1 small jalapeno, seeded and sliced

¼ cup onion, sliced

2 tablespoons diced plum or cherry tomato

⅓ cup vegan cheese shreds (pepper jack is really tasty!)

Directions:

Preheat the oven to 400 degrees, Fahrenheit and cover a baking sheet with foil. The foil makes the crust crispier.

Separate the English muffin and spread on some salsa and refried beans.

Place some of the jalapenos and onions on top and sprinkle the cheese over all.

Place on the baking sheet and bake for 10 to 15 minutes or until brown. You can turn on the broiler for a minute or two to melt the cheese.

Quinoa Trail Mix Cups

Preparation time: 5 minutes

Cooking time: 20 minutes

Servings: 4

Ingredients:

2 tablespoons ground flaxseed

⅓ cup unsweetened soy milk

1 cup old-fashioned rolled oats

1 cup cooked and cooled quinoa

¼ cup brown sugar

1 teaspoon ground cinnamon

¼ teaspoon salt

¼ cup pumpkin or sunflower seeds

¼ cup shredded coconut

½ cup almonds

½ cup raisins or dried cherries/cranberries

Directions:

Whisk the flaxseed and milk together in a small bowl and set aside for 10 minutes so the seed can absorb the milk.

Preheat the oven to 350 degrees, Fahrenheit and coat a muffin tin with coconut oil.

In a large bowl, mix the oats, quinoa, brown sugar, cinnamon, salt, pumpkin seeds, coconut, almonds and raisins.

Stir in the flaxseed and milk mixture and combine thoroughly.

Place two heaping teaspoons of the trail mix mixture in each muffin cup. When done, wet your fingers and press down on each muffin cup to compact the trail mix.

Bake for 12 minutes.

Cool completely before removing and each little cup will fall out. Store in an airtight container.

Sesame Potato Bites

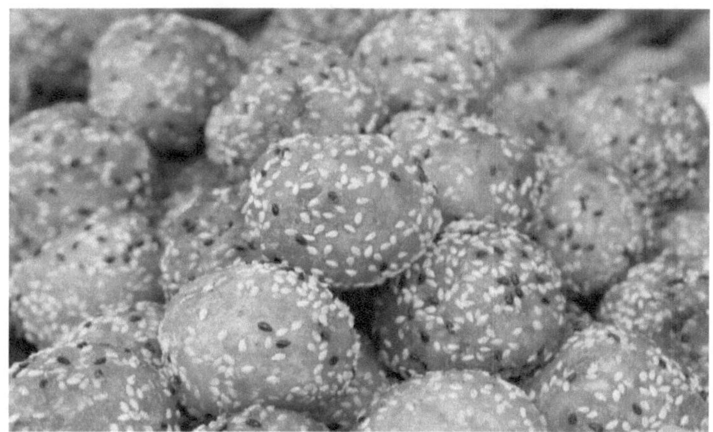

Preparation time: 5 minutes

Cooking time: 20 minutes

Servings: 4

Ingredients:

4 medium sized russet potatoes, washed and chopped, but not peeled

3 tablespoons olive oil, divided

3 cloves garlic, diced

1 cup onion, chopped

Salt and pepper to taste

¾ teaspoon baking powder

¼ cup nutritional yeast

½ cup potato starch

1 teaspoon salt

1 teaspoon paprika

⅛ teaspoon cayenne pepper

1 teaspoon dried oregano

¼ cup fresh parsley, finely chopped

1½ cups sesame seeds, even more as needed

Directions:

Place the potato pieces in a pot with enough water to cover them and bring to a boil.

Boil until the potatoes are soft and good for mashing.

Drain the potatoes, return them to the pot and mash by hand.

Add two tablespoons of the olive oil, along with the salt and pepper to taste; stir to mix. If the results are too thick, add a little water until they become creamy, then set them aside to cool.

Place the remaining olive oil in a skillet over medium high heat; add the garlic and onion and sauté for about three minutes, until the onion is soft. Add to the potato mixture and stir to combine.

Preheat the oven to 400 degrees, Fahrenheit and when potatoes are cool enough to handle, add the chickpea flour, baking powder, nutritional yeast, potato starch, salt, paprika, cayenne pepper, oregano and parsley and mix well. You should now have a dough that is much thicker than ordinary mashed potatoes.

Form the dough into golf-ball-sized spheres and roll in the sesame seeds. Place on a baking sheet covered with parchment paper and press down to flatten the balls a little.

Bake for 15 minutes, remove from the oven and flip each ball over, then return to the oven and bake for 15 more minutes.

Let the bites cool before serving.

Sweet Strawberry Fruit Leather

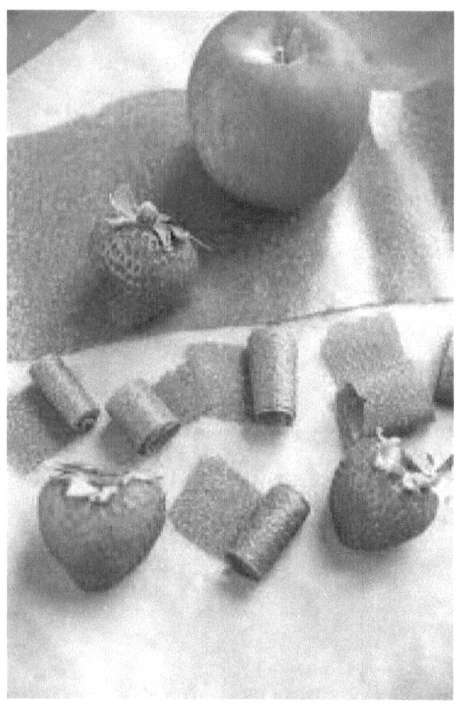

Preparation time: 5 minutes

Cooking time: 30 minutes

Servings: 4

Ingredients:

1½ pounds fresh s trawberries

½ cup sugar

3 tablespoons lemon juice

2 pinches of salt

Directions:

Preheat the oven to 170 degrees, Fahrenheit.

Place a silicone mat over a cookie sheet (you will need more than one). If you do not have silicone mats on hand, you can use oiled parchment paper, but the leather may still manage to stick to it.

Place the strawberries in a blender in batches and process until smooth. Pour the liquefied strawberries into a bowl.

Add the sugar, lemon juice and salt and stir to thoroughly combine.

Spread the mixture over the silicone sheet, leaving a space on each side so the leather is easily pulled off the mat when done.

Place the baking sheets in the oven and watch. The leather cooks slowly. The cooking process can take up to three hours. The mixture will be thick and pliable but will stick together and pull up from the pan. Let it cool before trying to pull it up or you will burn your fingers.

Pull up the sheet of fruit leather and place it on a cutting board. Use a pizza cutter to cut strips and place on a piece of parchment paper that is a little wider and longer than the strip. Roll the leather up along with the parchment paper.

Store your fruit leather in an airtight container until ready to eat.

Zucchini Chips

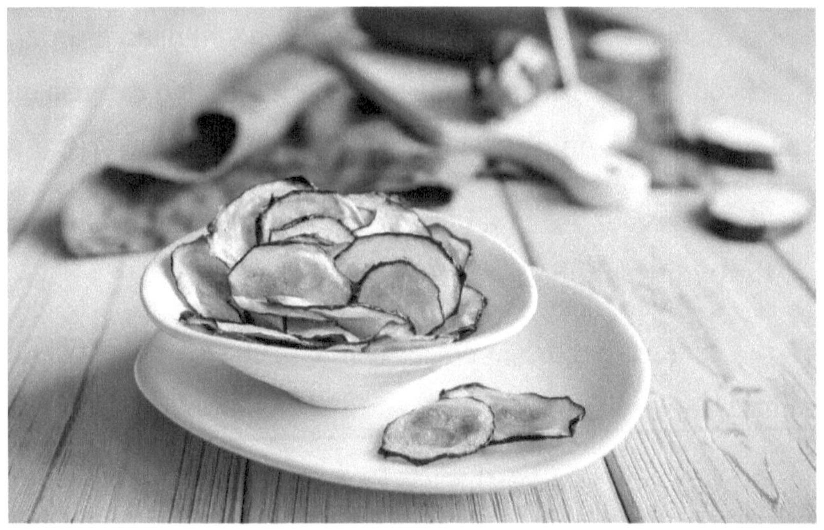

Preparation time: 5 minutes

Cooking time: 20 minutes

Servings: 4

Ingredients:

1 medium zucchini, thinly sliced with skin on

1 tablespoon olive oil

1 teaspoon salt

¼ teaspoon pepper

¾ teaspoon paprika

Directions:

Preheat the oven to 400 degrees, Fahrenheit and prepare two baking sheets with parchment paper.

Place the slices of zucchini on the baking sheets and make sure they are not touching.

Brush lightly with olive oil.

Mix the salt, pepper and paprika in a small bowl, whisking it together. Sprinkle on the zucchini chips.

Place in the oven and bake for 10 minutes. Rotate the pan and bake for 15 more minutes, watching to ensure that they don't scorch or turn too brown.

Let the chips cool for five minutes before serving.

Lemony Coconut Bars

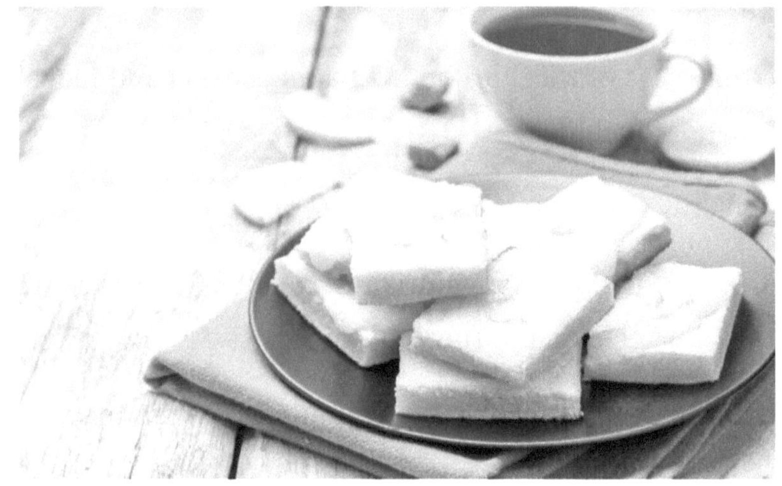

Preparation time: 5 minutes

Cooking time: 25 minutes

Servings: 4

Ingredients:

1 cup old-fashioned rolled oats

1½ cup unsweetened shredded coconut

2 tablespoons agave syrup

1 lemon

Directions:

Place the rolled oats in a food processor and pulse a few times, to grind them finely. Pour this into a mixing bowl.

Place the coconut in the food processor and pulse until it is mealy. Pour into the bowl with the oats.

Add the agave syrup, vanilla, coconut oil and oat flour; stir to mix.

Zest the lemon into the bowl.

Cut the lemon in half and squeeze both halves into the bowl.

Stir well. You should have a thick dough-like substance.

Press into a pan that has been lined with parchment paper. Refrigerate it for about two hours, until the mixture becomes slightly hardened. Cut into squares and serve.

Miniature Fruit Cheesecakes

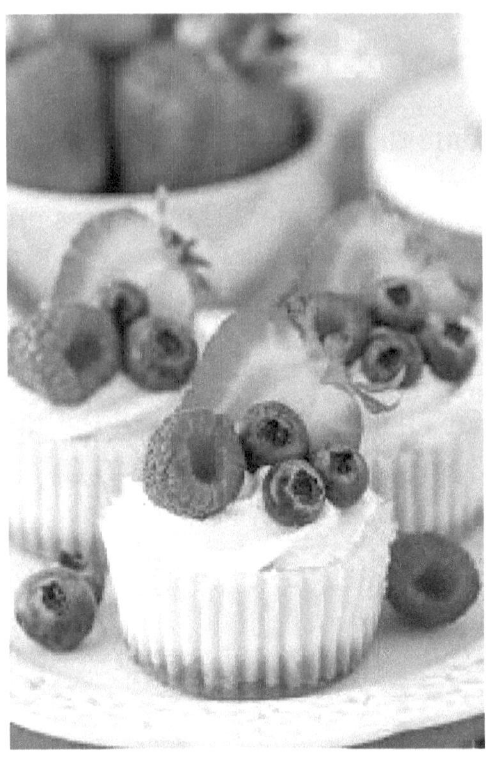

Preparation time: 5 minutes

Cooking time: 30 minutes

Servings: 4

Ingredients:

2 cups raw cashews soaked overnight in enough water to cover them

3 tablespoons old-fashioned rolled oats

1 cup pecans

1 tablespoon ground flaxseed

3 large dates with pits removed

½ teaspoon seal salt

1½ large lemons, both the zest and the juice

1 tablespoon coconut oil, melted

2 tablespoons maple syrup

1 tablespoon unsweetened almond milk

Fresh blueberries or raspberries for garnish

Directions:

Place the cashews in a bowl and cover with water. Cover with plastic wrap and set aside overnight.

Prepare a 12-hole muffin tin, placing cupcake liners in each hole.

In a food processor, place the oats, pecans, flaxseed, dates and salt; process until it forms a sticky dough.

Drop a level tablespoon of dough into the bottom of each cupcake liner and press down. Set the muffin tin aside.

Drain and rinse the cashews and put them in a high speed blender. Pulse to break them up. Add the juice from one lemon and the zest from that lemon. Save the zest from the half lemon for later. Add the coconut oil, maple syrup and almond milk; blend for about 90 seconds. Scrape down the sides and blend again until the mixture is thoroughly combined and looks smooth and creamy.

Use 1½ teaspoons of filling to complete each mini-cheesecake. Sprinkle with lemon zest and place a berry on top.

Refrigerate at least three hours before serving.

Minty Chocolate Chip Truffles

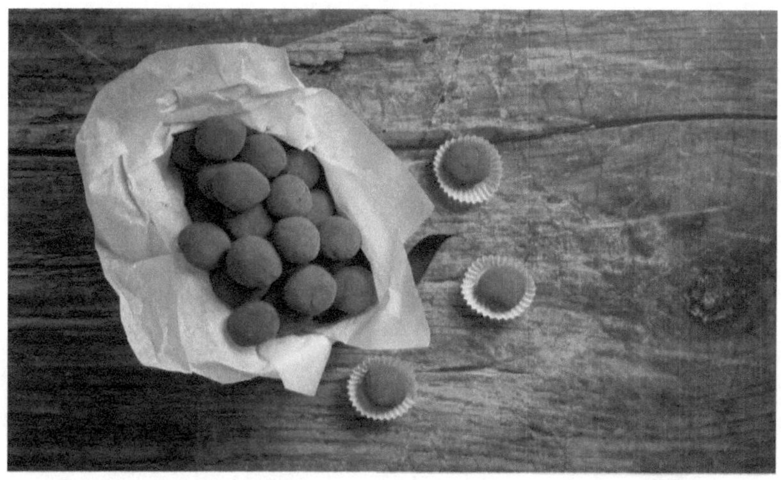

Preparation time: 5 minutes

Cooking time: 20 minutes

Servings: 4

Ingredients:

3 tablespoons mini chocolate chips

Cacao powder for dusting

Directions:

Place the peanut butter, applesauce and agave syrup in a mixing bowl; combine with a mixer.

Add the flour, about a quarter cup at a time and combine well.

Mix in the extract.

Stir in the chocolate chips by hand.

Roll the dough into about 12 one-inch balls and roll them in cacao powder to prevent stickiness. I like to refrigerate them for about an hour before serving.

They will keep well for three to five days refrigerated in an airtight container, that is, if they aren't devoured immediately.

No-bake Chocoholic Pie

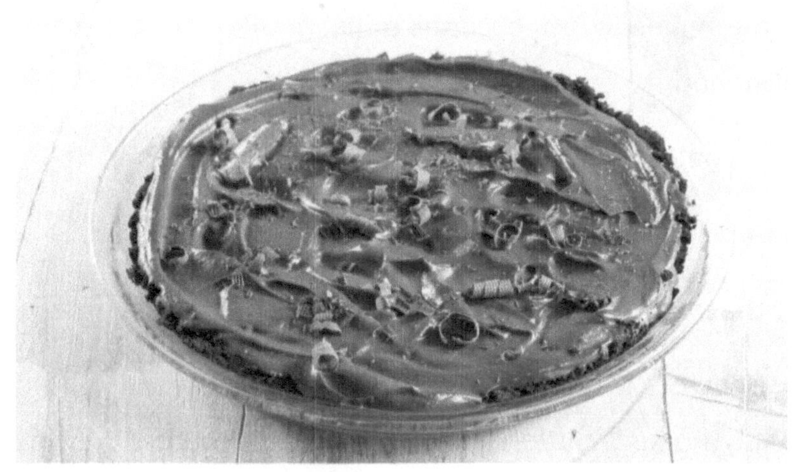

Preparation time: 5 minutes

Cooking time: 10 minutes

Servings: 4

Ingredients:

1 premade pie crust

1 pound silken tofu

3 tablespoons maple syrup

1 cup full-fat coconut milk

½ teaspoon salt

⅔ cup nondairy chocolate chips, melted

Directions:

Place the tofu in a blender and pulse to break it up.

Add the maple syrup, coconut milk, vanilla and salt, blending until smooth.

Remove one cup of the mixture for later.

Add the melted chocolate chips and blend them in well.

Pour the mixture from the blender into the prepared pie crust.

Pour a cup of the non-chocolate mixture on top and spread it out carefully. Take a butter knife and swirl it around to bring up some of the chocolate-infused mixture and create beautiful designs on top of the pie.

Refrigerate for at least two hours before serving.

No-bake Peanut Butter Chocolate Balls

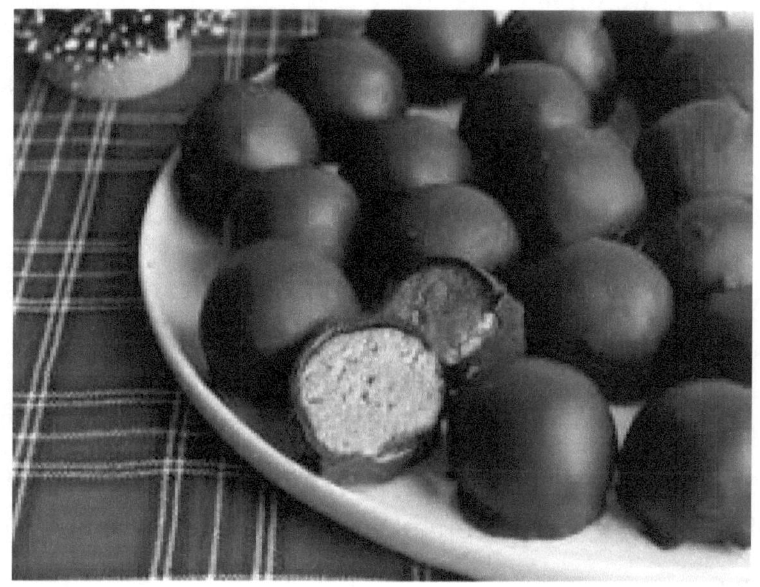

Preparation time: 5 minutes

Cooking time: 25minutes

Servings: 4

Ingredients:

1 cup pitted dates

¾ cups old-fashioned rolled oats

3 tablespoons peanut butter

¼ cup chocolate chips

Directions:

Place the dates in a bowl and cover them with warm water. Soak for about 15 minutes.

Drain the dates and use your hands to squeeze out any excess water; dry the dates on clean paper towels.

Place the dates in a food processor and roughly chop them.

Add the oats and peanut butter and pulse to form a sticky dough. Pour the dough into a bowl.

Fold in the chocolate chips and shape dough pieces into balls. Place them on a baking sheet lined with either wax paper or parchment paper. Refrigerate the balls for a few hours before serving.

Store in an airtight container in the refrigerator.

No-bake Pecan Apricot Balls

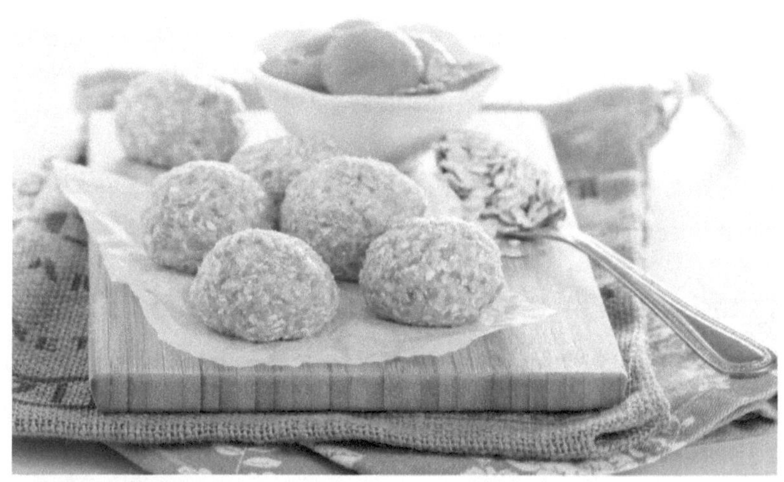

Preparation time: 5 minutes

Cooking time: 40 minutes

Servings: 4

Ingredients:

1 cup dried apricots

½ cup pecans

1 teaspoon vanilla extract

½ cup old-fashioned rolled oats

½ cup shredded coconut (optional)

Directions:

Place apricots in a food processor and pulse to chop until they are mealy.

Add the pecans and chop on high for about 20 seconds.

Add the vanilla and oats and process to a smooth dough, about 20 more seconds.

Scoop the dough by tablespoons and form into balls. Roll each ball in the coconut and place on a baking sheet lined with wax paper or parchment paper.

Refrigerate the balls for about two hours. After serving, store any leftovers in the refrigerator in an airtight container.

No-bake Pistachio Balls

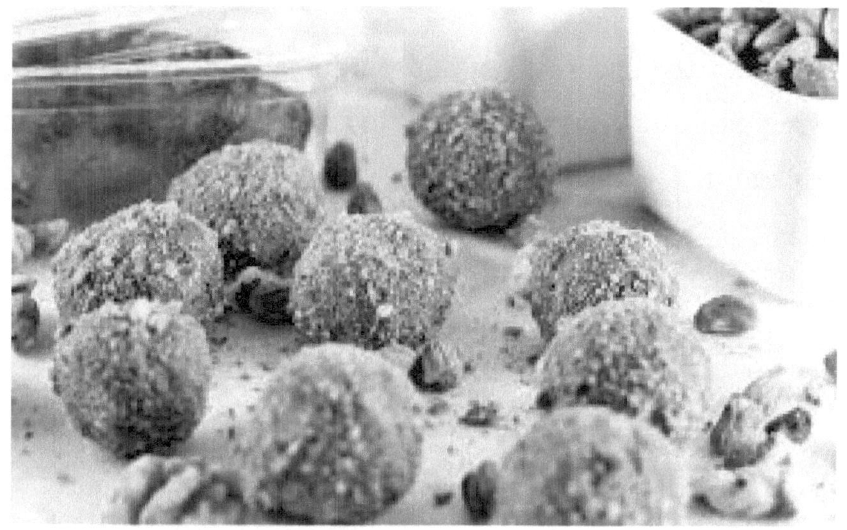

Preparation time: 5 minutes

Cooking time: 30 minutes

Servings: 4

Ingredients:

½ cup pistachio nuts, no shells

1 cup pitted dates

2 tablespoons coconut

Directions:

Place the pistachios in a food processor and chop well.

Add the dates and process until a dough forms.

Scoop out two tablespoons to make one ball, roll it in the coconut and place on baking sheet that's been lined with wax paper or parchment paper.

Refrigerate the sheet-full of cookies for about an hour before serving. Store any leftover cookies in an airtight container in the refrigerator.

Peach Crisp with Date Sugar

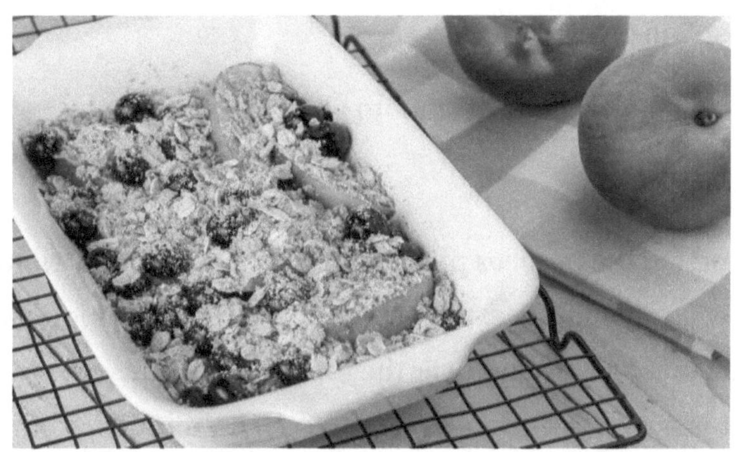

Preparation time: 5 minutes

Cooking time: 40 minutes

Servings: 4

Ingredients:

5 to 6 large peaches, peeled and sliced

3 tablespoons chia seeds

1 tablespoon lemon juice

3 teaspoons ground cinnamon, divided

⅛ cup date sugar

¼ cup oat flour

1 cup old-fashioned oats

½ additional cup date sugar

1 tablespoon maple syrup

⅛ teaspoon ground nutmeg

3 heaping tablespoons of smooth almond butter

Directions:

Peel and cut the peaches putting them in a bowl and sprinkle the chia seeds, lemon juice, two teaspoons of the cinnamon and the eighth cup of date sugar over the top. Give it a stir, taste to make sure it is sweet enough and set aside for 15 minutes so the chia seeds can thicken up.

Preheat the oven to 350 degrees, Fahrenheit.

Pour the peaches into the bottom of a nonstick sprayed 8½ by 11 inch baking dish and set aside.

In a bowl, prepare the topping by adding together the oat flour, rolled oats, half-cup of date sugar, maple syrup, the remaining teaspoon of cinnamon, the nutmeg and the almond butter and mixing well. It should have a crumbly consistency.

Sprinkle the crumb mixture on top of the peaches.

Bake for 30 minutes or until the topping browns. Let it cool for 10 minutes before serving.

Pumpkin Oatmeal Cookies

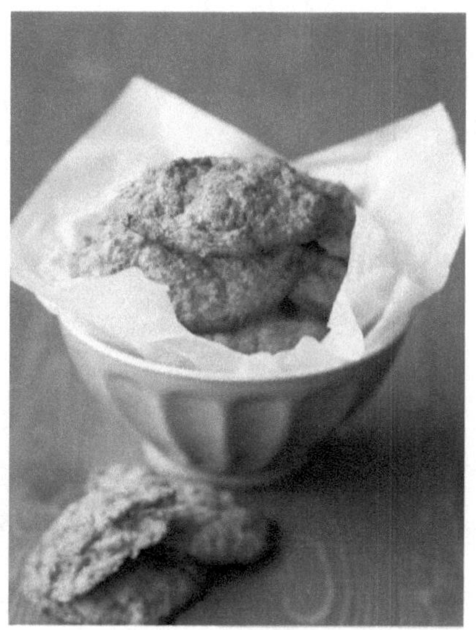

Preparation time: 5 minutes

Cooking time: 20 minutes

Servings: 4

Ingredients:

1 cup oat flour

2 cups old-fashioned rolled oats

1 cup sugar or ½ cup date sugar

1 teaspoon baking soda

¼ teaspoon nutmeg

1 teaspoon cinnamon

⅛ teaspoon salt

1 15-ounce can pumpkin puree

¼ cup vanilla almond milk

½ cup golden raisins (optional)

Directions:

Preheat the oven to 35 degrees, Fahrenheit and cover two baking sheets with parchment paper.

Place the oat flour, rolled outs, sugar, baking soda, nutmeg, cinnamon and salt in a large mixing bowl and stir together.

Combine the puree and the almond milk and whisk together.

Pour the pumpkin puree mixture into the dry mixture, stirring well with a wooden spoon after each addition. Once it is well mixed, add the raisins if you are going to use them.

Scoop the batter out, a heaping tablespoon at a time and roll it into a ball. Space these balls apart evenly on the baking sheets.

Flatten each ball lightly with a fork.

Bake for 24 to 28 minutes, until brown. Let the cookies cool for five minutes before transferring them to cooling racks.

Raspberry Fudge Tart

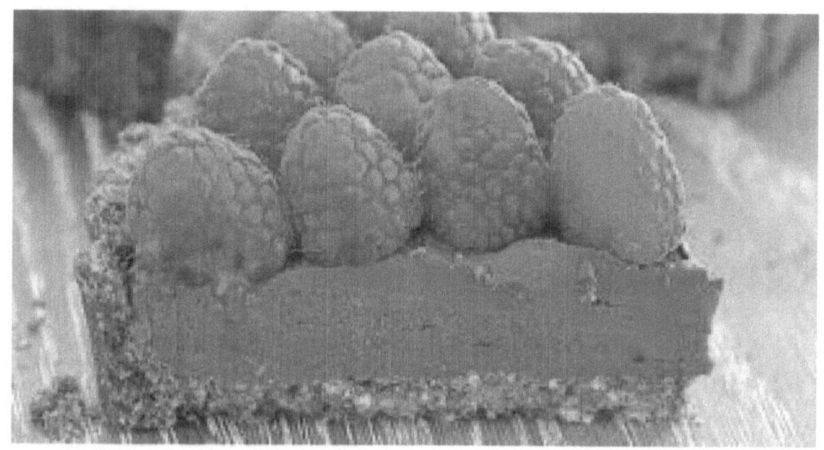

Preparation time: 5 minutes

Cooking time: 50 minutes

Servings: 4

Ingredients for crust:

2 cups old-fashioned roll ed oats

1 tablespoon coconut sugar

4 tablespoons cocoa

¼ cup coconut oil

¼ teaspoon salt

5 to 7 tablespoons cold water

Ingredients for filling:

2 cups canned chickpeas, rinsed and drained well

2 tablespoons coconut oil

5 tablespoons cocoa

½ cup semi-sweet dark chocolate chips

½ teaspoon salt

6 tablespoons maple syrup

1 tablespoon vanilla extract

4 tablespoons almond milk

1 large container of fresh raspberries

Directions:

Preheat the oven to 350 degrees, Fahrenheit and coat a tart pan with nonstick spray, then set aside.

Place the oats in a food processor or blender and process until they become a coarse flour.

Add the coconut sugar, cocoa, coconut oil and salt; process until combined.

Gradually add the water, one tablespoon at a time. Check after the third tablespoon. If the dough sticks together when you squeeze it with your hands, it is ready. If not, keep adding water until it does.

Press the dough into the tart pan on the bottom and up the sides evenly; prick the dough with a fork.

Take a piece of parchment paper and set it on top of the crust. Pour dried beans on top of the parchment paper to weight down the crust. Bake it for 25 minutes.

Remove the beans and the paper, then return the crust to the oven for 10 more minutes. Remove it and wait until the crust is completely cool before adding the filling.

Place the rinsed and drained chickpeas in the food processor and pulse to break them up.

Add the coconut oil, cocoa, chocolate chips, salt, maple syrup, vanilla and milk; process until smooth.

Pour this mixture into the crust and top with raspberries.

Place in the refrigerator for at least two hours before serving.

Strawberry Pie with Walnut Crust

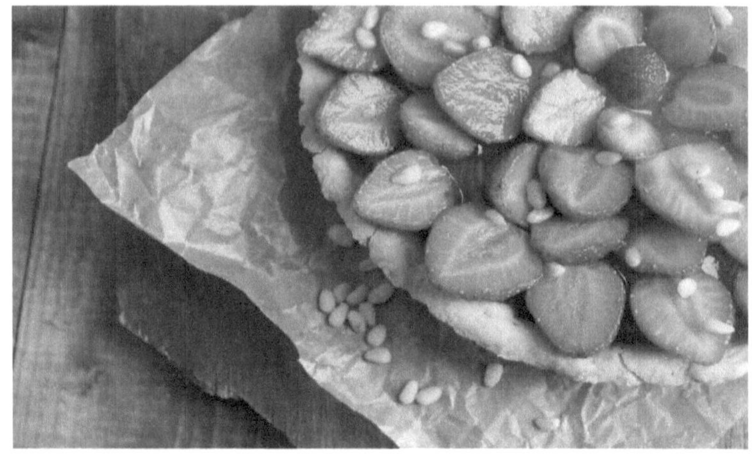

Preparation time: 5 minutes

Cooking time: 20 minutes

Servings: 4

Ingredients:

¾ cup raw walnuts

1 cup oat flour

¾ cups rolled oats

¼ teaspoon Himalayan salt (optional: substitute regular table salt)

3 tablespoons maple syrup

¼ cup coconut oil, melted

2½ pounds fresh strawberries, divided

2 tablespoons cornstarch

¼ cup water

½ cup apple juice

3 tablespoons turbinado sugar

Directions:

Preheat oven to 350 degrees, Fahrenheit and coat a deep dish pie pan with nonstick spray.

Place the walnuts in the food processor and pulse until they are roughly chopped with no large chunks.

Add the oat flour, the rolled oats, salt, maple syrup and melted coconut oil; pulse until everything is well combined.

Pour the mixture into the pie pan and gently press it down on the bottom and up the sides.

Bake the crust for 10 to 15 minutes or until the edges brown. Remove from the oven and set the pan on a cooling rack.

Take six strawberries and remove the stems. Put them in a blender and liquefy them. Pour into a quarter-cup measuring cup and if you do not have enough to make a fourth of a cup, liquefy a few more until you do. If you have a little more than a fourth cup, it will not matter. Pour this strawberry puree into a small saucepan.

In a small bowl, combine the cornstarch and the water. Stir until the cornstarch is dissolved.

Place the saucepan over medium heat and add the apple juice and the sugar. Whisk well and bring the contents to a simmer.

Once it starts to boil, reduce the heat to a simmer and whisk constantly until it turns shiny and thickens to form a glaze. Remove from the heat and set aside.

Hull and slice the rest of the strawberries into a bowl and pour the glaze over the top. Gently fold the glaze in and pour it all into the baked pie crust.

Refrigerate for 45 minutes to an hour before slicing and serving.

Conclusion

To survive, we need to eat. As a result, food has turned into a symbol of loving, nurturing and sharing with one another. Recording, collecting, sharing and remembering the recipes that have been passed to you by your family is a great way to immortalize and honor your family. It is these traditions that carve out your individual personality. You will not just be honoring your family tradition by cooking these recipes, but they will also inspire you to create your own variations, which you can then pass on to your children's.

Diets are mostly confusing and not clear for people in general. Everyone who starts a diet plan has to face issues with the nutritional value, overall immunity among other things as well. All these issues come on the surface due to a lack of awareness and research. The eBook explains all the necessary points, guidelines and recipes for the plant-based diet plan. It is a complete help for those who do not want to miss anything in their diet and get the maximum benefits.

By following the plant based diet, You are going to feel better. You are going to improve your mood and energy levels. If you have been battling mental health problems, then using the plant-based diet is going to help you work on those problems.

The recipes are just passed on to everyone, and nobody actually possesses them. I too love sharing recipes. The collection is vibrant and rich as a number of home cooks have offered their inputs to ensure that all of us can cook delicious meals at our home. I am thankful to each one of you who has contributed to this book and has allowed their traditions to pass on and grow with others. You guys are wonderful!

At the end of this cookbook, here are quick tips for you that will help you get most out of the plant-based diet. Increase the use of whole foods in your diet. It is stable already at breakfast for most people but also utilize them whenever possible as they provide much-needed carbs and energy. Eating oatmeal for breakfast is a good start in following this diet.

www.ingramcontent.com/pod-product-compliance
Lightning Source LLC
Chambersburg PA
CBHW051437250726
48655CB00001B/102